"The end to digestive distress begins with a thorough reading of *The Whol-* _____ This clear, concise, and elegant book e_____ n of gut pain and suffering in a way ev_____ v. The recipe section is a delight, w_____ nourishing dishes and meal plans. Th_____ ."

—Edward Bauman, M.Ed., Ph.D, director of
Bauman College: Holistic Nutrition and Culinary
Arts in Berkeley, CA

"As a nutrition expert, I see clients on a regular basis who have digestive issues. I am thrilled to have Laura Knoff's book to refer them to. It is a great resource for anyone suffering from digestive issues or wanting to improve their overall health and vitality. Laura's style is easy to understand and, more importantly, simple to implement. Everyone would benefit by following the concepts in this book."

—JJ Virgin, Ph.D., CNS, author of *Six Weeks to
Sleeveless and Sexy*

"Knoff brings us a book that will help outsmart disruptive digestive discomforts once and for all. The delicious recipes provided in her book will be embraced by the entire family. I highly recommend this book for everybody who needs easy strategies and solutions for soothing the gastrointestinal tract."

—Ann Louise Gittleman, Ph.D., CNS, bestselling
author of *Fat Flush Plan* and *Fat Flush for Life*

THE

WHOLE-FOOD GUIDE TO
Overcoming Irritable Bowel Syndrome

STRATEGIES & RECIPES FOR EATING WELL WITH IBS, INDIGESTION & OTHER DIGESTIVE DISORDERS

LAURA J. KNOFF, NC

New Harbinger Publications, Inc.

Distributed in Canada by Raincoast Books

Copyright © 2010 by Laura Knoff, B.Sc.,
New Harbinger Publications, Inc.
5674 Shattuck Avenue
Oakland, CA 94609
www.newharbinger.com

FSC
Mixed Sources
Product group from well-managed
forests and other controlled sources
Cert no. SW-COC-002283
www.fsc.org
© 1996 Forest Stewardship Council

Acquired by Jess O'Brien; Cover design by Amy Shoup;
Edited by Nelda Street; Text design by Michele Waters-Kermes

Library of Congress Cataloging-in-Publication Data

Knoff, Laura J.
  The whole-food guide to overcoming irritable bowel syndrome : strategies and recipes for eating well with IBS, indigestions, and other digestive disorders / Laura J. Knoff.
    p. cm.
  Includes bibliographical references and index.
  ISBN 978-1-57224-798-7
  1. Irritable colon--Popular works. 2. Irritable colon--Diet therapy--Popular works. I. Title.
  RC862.I77K56 2010
  616.3'42--dc22
                        2010009834

12   11   10

10   9   8   7   6   5   4   3   2   1   First printing

Acknowledgments and Dedication

I wish to thank my parents for nurturing my curiosity and problem-solving abilities, my editors, mentors, teachers, clients, and students who are also my teachers. I especially want to thank my Diana, who has supplied unwavering support in so many ways.

Contents

Introduction

In the United States alone, 10 to 15 percent of the population—45.5 million people—suffers from irritable bowel syndrome (IBS) (Saito, Schoenfeld, and Locke 2002). If you are among them, I wrote this book to help you take charge of your life and work toward regaining your health. I want to provide you with some tools to help you find the best diet for you, and I'd like to share what worked for me in my healing process, so you and others can learn from my experience of overcoming IBS without drugs or surgery. Through careful observation and alternative testing, I was able to discover what foods, environmental factors, pathogens (such as harmful bacteria, viruses, and fungi), activities, and emotions contributed to my IBS symptoms. I was able to address the pathogens and change my eating and lifestyle habits. Once I changed my diet, my digestion improved in two weeks. As I continued incorporating lifestyle changes and repairing my gut, the symptoms slowly and consistently subsided. Today my digestion is healed, and if I have a minor upset, I can identify the source and recover in hours instead of months. I don't take any drugs, and I take only a few specific supplements, which I'll identify for you.

After healing my own digestion with whole foods, relaxation, massage, gentle exercise, herbs, and supplements, I became a certified nutrition consultant, and I have helped many others improve their overall digestion and overcome IBS. I hope this book will give you the tools to help you find the solution to your own IBS.

With the information in this book, I hope to help you answer these questions:

- What is IBS, and how do I know if I have it?

- How is the digestive system supposed to work?

- What's likely to contribute to IBS?

- How do I figure out what's making my gut hurt and what to do about it?

- How do I choose foods that won't give me pain, and why do some whole foods help?

- What does stress have to do with it?

- What about fiber?

- Are there herbs or supplements that will help?

- What do I eat?

- Can I ever eat out again?

You can find the answers to these questions by following this book step by step. If you use the forms this book provides to document your own reactions to foods and activities, you'll begin to notice what affects your digestion and overall health. Follow the simple recipes and use them as starting points to fine-tune your diet. Be patient with yourself. Regaining proper bowel function and healing yourself can take time. Do the best you can and realize that no one's perfect. If you have a relapse, don't agonize; instead, analyze and learn what you need to do differently next time. Even slow progress is beneficial and indicates healing. I'm living proof that healing is not only possible but also likely, if you give yourself the attention and care you deserve. Your body wants to be whole and healthy, and if you give it the opportunity, that's what you can expect.

The most effective approach to any health challenge is to look at the entire body, lifestyle, and attitude in order to change the process of degeneration to one of regeneration. Everything affects everything else. Our digestive system is a continuous unit that is attached to, and interacts with, the rest of the body. Each part of the digestive system depends on all the other parts. Gulping our food without thoroughly chewing it results in an irritated intestine. The chemicals we encounter in our food and environment as part of our modern life can irritate the entire gut tube, not just the area of entry. This is because we can eat chemicals, inhale them, or absorb them through the skin. Also, spending excess energy worrying can deplete energy needed to repair or maintain our digestive process, potentially resulting in IBS. The key is to proceed with awareness and attention to the food you eat and how you eat it, and to simplify your overall environment. This holistic approach can help you regain a healthy life, free of IBS.

CHAPTER 1

Name It and Claim It

Irritable bowel syndrome (IBS), sometimes called *spastic colon* or *nervous indigestion*, is one of twenty-five functional gastrointestinal disorders (Olden 1996). It can be severe enough to prevent you from working or leaving home, lest a toilet be too far away. Defined by its symptoms after other possible causes are eliminated, IBS is characterized as: abdominal pain or cramping relieved by a bowel movement; changes in bowel habits; stool urgency; diarrhea, constipation, or both; and gas and bloating in the absence of detectable structural abnormalities or other causes (Bolen 2009). Many of the symptoms of IBS also apply to inflammatory bowel disease (IBD), celiac disease, and cancer, so it's important to consult a medical doctor to rule out these serious diseases (Collins 1994).

POSSIBLE CAUSES AND MISSED DIAGNOSES

The most often overlooked cause of IBS, *celiac disease* is an inherited sensitivity to *gluten*, the protein in wheat and other cereal grains. Celiac disease is an extreme enough autoimmune disease to potentially destroy the intestinal lining. Two studies showed that 10 percent of participants with IBS had celiac disease (Shahbazkhani et al. 2003; Sanders et al. 2001). Doctors use antibody testing of blood and saliva samples to diagnose celiac disease, and genetic testing (by mouth swab) can determine if you are predisposed to it, even if you no longer consume gluten.

Doctors' gold standard for diagnosing celiac disease is to use a biopsy to look for damage to the small intestine. But since the intestine can heal itself in a matter of months, if you didn't consume gluten at all for several weeks prior to the biopsy, you could get false-negative results. A false negative means that little or no damage was found. Some doctors still believe there must be total destruction of the villi of the small intestine to diagnose celiac disease, but newer data shows that even partial villi destruction indicates celiac disease (O'Bryan 2008).

When you are trying to overcome IBS, you need to ask what's irritating your gut. The answer could be nearly anything, from various food allergens or chemicals to an imbalance of gut flora to hormone and neurotransmitter imbalances (Talley 2006). The same substances that cause the intestine to spasm and quickly eliminate the bowel's contents can sometimes lead to more serious conditions if the cause is not addressed, or if drugs or laxatives, which thwart the body's protective and self-healing mechanisms, are used.

The problem with IBS is that the actual cause of the symptoms may be overlooked or downplayed as stress, or you might even hear your doctor say something like, "It's all in your head." Many people with real but undetected causes of abdominal discomfort have been given antidepressants or tranquilizers to reduce their pain (Waxman 1988). The key word is "undetected." As we get better at finding a cause for this type of irritation, it's likely that there will be fewer IBS diagnoses. In many of my clients, a specialized stool test not only shows the presence of pathogenic or imbalanced bacteria in the gut (also known as *dysbiosis*), but also indicates how well the digestive system is working (Goldberg, Trivieri, and Anderson 2002). Specialized laboratories test for antibodies to specific pathogens and can indicate which treatments are most effective (see the resources for a list of laboratories). *Colonoscopy*, or endoscopic examination of the colon, shows only structural issues, not microscopic changes or bacterial infection. Once the pathogen is eliminated or the imbalance corrected, the gut can heal, and IBS symptoms can disappear.

It's becoming well known that people with IBD, such as Crohn's disease or ulcerative colitis, often also have IBS. The difference between IBS and IBD is that people with IBD have detectable structural abnormalities (Collins 1994). I think of IBS as one of the first steps on the continuum of dysfunctional digestion. IBS may also be just one symptom of a life out of balance. IBS affects the whole body and mind, and vice versa.

Not knowing when they will need a toilet can cause many IBS sufferers to restrict their activities considerably. The inability to feel comfortable in your own body can be depressing and anxiety producing. When you can't rely on your digestion, what can you rely on? Food can become the enemy. You may find it easier to eat little, since many symptoms are reduced or eliminated when the digestive system isn't called on to do any work. Some foods may not cause symptoms for a while, but, due to overconsumption, may start triggering symptoms later, further narrowing the variety of foods you can eat.

When something irritates another part of our body, we avoid it. We can physically move away from and avoid a skin irritant. We can wash away bacteria and irritating chemicals, such as paint or poison oak sap. We can avoid insects or swat them away to protect our skin. Similarly, we can eliminate an irritant from the digestive tract; the body uses sudden diarrhea (and sometimes vomiting) to get rid of the toxic irritants excreted by some pathogenic bacteria, such as those involved in food poisoning. Some other microbial toxins (like those produced by *Clostridium difficile*) directly alter the rate of bowel movement less violently (Joneja 2004). If the body succeeds at eliminating the pathogen, there's no resulting infection, since the intestinal contents are actually part of the exterior environment, not part of our tissues.

Unfortunately, though, we may not be able to directly identify the digestive tract irritant, because it may be from something we consumed days before, or it may relate to something we breathe (chemical exposure) or even to the hormones we produce during stress, monthly cycles, or both. We can't avoid an irritant we can't identify, so we keep coming in contact with it. And just as a continuous skin irritation can lead to inflammation and disease of the skin, the same applies to an ongoing irritation of the internal "skin" of the digestive system. Continuing to eat foods or substances that cause reactions, and that our bowels then try to reject, may eventually make us tolerate those foods—but damage continues to occur. If we ignore the warning signs, the unchecked causes can eventually lead to damage and a more severe diagnosis.

The key to keeping food from becoming the enemy, it turns out, is to vary your diet every day on a four-day rotation plan. I'll show you how to identify and avoid your trigger foods, and help you set up a rotation diet to prevent your body from reacting to replacement foods.

HOW DO I KNOW IF I HAVE IBS?

No specific test exists for IBS, so ruling out other diseases and physical causes is the first step. The primary symptom is chronic abdominal pain, often very severe, possibly accompanied by a bowel movement or relieved after a bowel movement. The Rome Foundation is a nonprofit organization that helps those with functional gastrointestinal disorders. They use the following criteria to diagnose IBS. If you have two of the following symptoms, your abdominal pain may be associated with IBS (Longstreth et al. 2006):

- Pain relief with defecation

- Onset of pain or discomfort associated with change in frequency of stool

- Onset of pain or discomfort associated with change in form of stool

Several variations (subtypes) of IBS exist, and though they are not absolute, one or more of the symptoms of a subtype must be present to identify that specific subtype (Mearin et al. 2003):

1. Diarrhea-predominant IBS (IBS-D)

    - three or more bowel movements a day

    - loose, watery stools

    - fecal urgency

2. Constipation-predominant IBS (IBS-C)

    - fewer than three bowel movements a week

    - hard or lumpy stools

    - straining during bowel movements

3. Mixed-type IBS (IBS-M)

    - both hard and loose stools over a period of hours or days

4. Alternating-type IBS (IBS-A)

    - change from one subtype to another over periods of weeks or months

Other symptoms you may experience with IBS include:

- whitish mucus in the stool

- swollen or bloated abdomen

- incomplete evacuation (the feeling that you haven't finished a bowel movement)

Women with IBS often have more symptoms during the menstrual period. According to the American College of Gastroenterology, 80 percent of people with IBS are women (American College of Gastroenterology Functional Gastrointestinal Disorders Task Force 2002). About half of people with fibromyalgia or chronic fatigue syndrome are likely to have IBS (Blanchard and Abrams Brill 2004). Having an autoimmune condition also increases the risk of IBS, and vice versa (Ibid.). Interestingly, temporomandibular joint (TMJ) dysfunction is another common condition among IBS sufferers (Whitehead, Palsson, and Jones 2002). Muscle tension in the jaw may indicate stress, which also affects digestion and elimination, and TMJ may also affect chewing, which, as we'll see, is critical for good digestion.

I've created the following questionnaire for you to use in assessing your symptoms to see if you have IBS. Look back at your symptoms over the past six months (including your toilet habits). Rate the frequency of your symptoms and place the corresponding number in the table. When you've finished, add up the columns. Don't worry if you can't figure exactly how often you have the symptom; approximate. All of these symptoms are signs of disordered digestion, but some are more serious than others.

Scoring Key:

Never = 0

Less than once a week = 1

Once a week = 2

Many times a week = 3

Every day = 5

Many times a day = 7

SELF-ASSESSMENT QUESTIONNAIRE: HOW IS YOUR DIGESTION?

Symptoms of IBS	Score 0–7
Abdominal pain	
Alternating diarrhea and constipation	
Black stool*	
Bloating	
Bowel movement relieves abdominal pain	
Burping frequently	
Constipation	
Cramping	
Diarrhea or watery stool	
Feeling of incomplete evacuation	
Fewer than one stool a day	
Flatulence relieves abdominal pain	
Food visible in stool	
Foul-smelling stool or flatulence	
Excessive gas or flatulence	
Greasy stool or oil slick in toilet	
Green stool	
Gurgling noises in belly	
Hard, dry, or pellet stool	
Loose or soft stool	
More than three stools a day	
Mucus on stool or on toilet paper	
Pale- or light-colored stool	
Recent or frequent food poisoning or stomach flu	

Straining to pass a stool	
Symptoms worse during menstrual periods	
Thin or ribbon-shaped stool*	
Urgency to have a bowel movement	
Total Score	

*If you have this symptom, see your health care provider immediately.

Interpreting Your Score:

1 to 10   IBS is unlikely, but your digestion is not optimal.

11 to 25   IBS is possible. Simple changes may improve your symptoms within a short period.

26 to 50   IBS is probable. Follow this book's recommendations.

51 to 198   Consult a doctor. If disease is ruled out, you will likely be diagnosed with IBS. Following this book's suggestions will help you.

If you score over 50 and have been diagnosed with any of the conditions in the next table, you may need to seek help from a specialist in digestive disorders. If you hear "there's no cause" and you will "have to live with it," read on and follow this book's suggestions. There *are* causes and you don't have to live with the debilitating symptoms of IBS. You can do a lot to change your life for the better.

Check (√) all the following diagnoses that apply to you:

I have been diagnosed with...	
Chronic fatigue	
Fibromyalgia	
Chronic pelvic pain	
Temporomandibular joint dysfunction (TMJ)	

HOW IS THE DIGESTIVE SYSTEM SUPPOSED TO WORK?

We all eat. We think little about our digestion unless it's not working properly. Even as infants, we knew when we were hungry. As children, we learned what it felt like when we needed to poop and to control that need until we could get to a toilet. We also knew if our tummy hurt or if we didn't feel well, though as children, we may have had difficulty expressing that information. Beyond hunger or the need to defecate, most of us have no idea how our digestion should function. Improperly working digestion may result in IBS.

I Think, Therefore I Eat

Let's start at the beginning—with the brain, because it controls much of our digestive response, and it can enhance or reduce our ability to digest properly. We respond to thinking of, seeing, or smelling food by secreting saliva and other digestive juices. The food industry is well aware of this response and takes advantage of it, using advertising to entice people to consume its products as often as possible. Constantly being surrounded by food affects the digestive system's functionality. Digestion may overrespond or underrespond. People who are incessantly exposed to food or its images may succumb to overeating, or may consciously ignore urges to eat. Continuous consumption can tire your digestive process, cause excessive weight gain, or both. From my clinical experience with food-service workers, chefs, and waitpersons, ignoring hunger signals can confuse your natural digestive responses, reducing appetite and hunger awareness.

Aside from having a role in appetite, the brain plays a part in controlling blood flow, and thus digestive maintenance and repair. When we are calm, relaxed, and unrushed, the digestive system can easily provide the chemical secretions and muscular movements required to take food apart and extract what we need, as well as easily eliminate wastes, because blood circulation to the digestive system is properly maintained when we are relaxed. When we are stressed, circulation is partially diverted away from the digestive organs to the large muscles, heart, and lungs (Selye 1956).

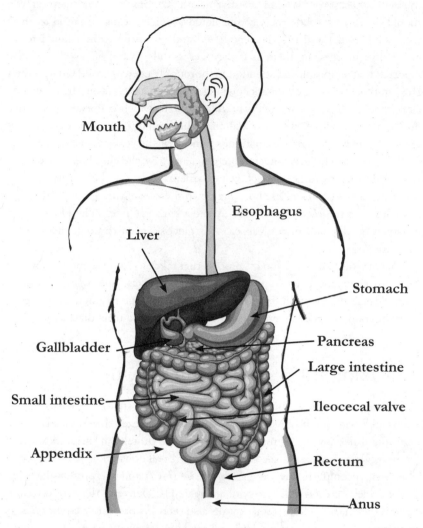

Figure 1.1   The Digestive System

Chew, Chew, Chew

In the mouth, your saliva secretions lubricate food as you chew, beginning the digestive process. Although it consists mostly of water, saliva also contains the enzymes *amylase* (to break down carbohydrates) and small amounts of *lipase* (to begin breaking down fats). Unless they are adequately mixed with the food through chewing, these enzymes have little or no effect, so careful and complete chewing is necessary for good digestive health. To improve your digestion, you should drink your solids and eat your liquids, which means you need to chew your solid foods until they become liquid and you need to mix liquid foods with saliva by chewing them as if they were solids. Many of my clients have reported that simply paying attention to thoroughly chewing food reduced their IBS symptoms. Eating on the run, gulping food, and eating faster than everyone else are all signs that you aren't chewing enough, which can lead to digestive problems. As we chew, we break and mash the food into small particles, allowing saliva enzymes to interact with much more of the surface area of the food. Well-chewed food digests much more efficiently. By chewing bread or cooked rice until it begins to taste sweet, you experience how starches transform into sugars, which is from amylase breaking down the carbohydrate bonds, allowing the release of the *glucose* that makes up most carbohydrates. The bloodstream can then quickly and directly absorb this glucose, even through the mouth's capillaries.

You then swallow the food, a process that takes it from the mouth down to the stomach via muscular contractions of the esophagus. The *esophageal sphincter*, a muscle near the top of the stomach, opens to allow food to enter, and closes to keep the food and acidic secretions inside the stomach during digestion.

Mixing It Up, Breaking It Down

Once in the stomach, the food mixes with more digestive secretions. Imagine a muscular bag, about the size of your fist, that squeezes the swallowed food, churning it like a washing machine, allowing the proteins to break down into amino acids and releasing the fats for further breakdown. The stomach secretions that accomplish this are *hydrochloric acid* (*HCl*) and the protein-digesting pre-enzyme *pepsinogen*. The acidity of adequate HCl converts the pepsinogen to its active form, *pepsin*. The stomach walls also secrete a protective layer of mucus to prevent the strongly acidic HCl and enzymes from digesting the stomach walls. In this acidic environment, protein foods, such as chicken or fish, break down, to be reconstructed as our own proteins later, in the liver.

HCl acts as an important health protector by killing harmful microbes that incoming food may contain. HCl also acts to dissolve minerals in the food, such as iron, calcium, magnesium, and zinc, allowing them to be easily absorbed. Ulcers are the result of too little mucus production and, often, weak HCl production, allowing a type of bacteria, *Helicobacter pylori* (*H. pylori*), to proliferate and destroy the stomach lining. *H. pylori* secretes ammonia, further reducing the acidic environment so it can flourish. When the stomach isn't acidic enough, food goes undigested and, instead, ferments. Fermentation in the stomach creates many problems, including excessive gas (burping or belching) and heart-burn, and can contribute to IBS (Joneja 2004).

Soaking It Up

Once the proteins enter the stomach, the hormone *gastrin* is secreted into the bloodstream. Gastrin stimulates an increase in acid production, the stomach's muscular contractions, and pancreatic secretions. The liquid mixture of partially digested food and secretions (called *chyme*) is released from the stomach into the first part of the small intestine by the pyloric sphincter's opening and closing. A series of muscular contractions and relaxations, called *peristalsis*, initiates the transport of the chyme along the digestive system's entire length.

Though only about an inch in diameter, the small intestine is about twenty-one feet long. The small intestine's entire interior surface is lined with tiny fingerlike projections, called *villi*, which selectively absorb nutrients once the digestive process has made them small enough. Because these many villi cover the small intestine's length, its surface area averages twenty-four hundred square feet, or slightly larger than a singles tennis court but smaller than a basketball court (Brynie 2002). That huge amount of surface area is necessary for us to digest and absorb as much as possible from our food. You can better understand this when you consider that, ideally, food spends only eighteen to twenty-four hours in your digestive tract.

The small intestine consists of three parts: the duodenum, the jejunum, and the ileum. The first twelve inches makes up the *duodenum* (from Latin for "twelve"). Food continues to deconstruct along the duodenum, aided by several more enzyme secretions. The duodenum's villi produce important enzymes to break down *lactose* (milk sugar), *sucrose* (table sugar), and *maltose* (sugar from grains, malt, and starch). Made in the liver and stored in the gallbladder, *bile*—along with enzymes and bicarbonate from the pancreas—adds to the chyme in the duodenum via the common bile duct. Bile helps break fats into very small droplets to allow the fat-digesting enzyme (lipase) secreted by the pancreas to break them into absorbable fatty acids and glycerol. Other enzymes, also made in the pancreas, further break down proteins, fats, and carbohydrates. The final actions of digestion continue along the next ten feet of small intestine, called the *jejunum*. The end result of this enzyme action is that *macronutrients* (amino acids, fatty acids, and glucose) and *micronutrients* (vitamins and minerals) that the food contains are primarily absorbed in the small intestine, with some minerals and water being absorbed in the large intestine.

Some absorption occurs all along the small intestine, but most happens in the *ileum*, the last ten feet. The ileum joins the large intestine, also known as the *colon* (large in diameter but only five feet in length, on average), at the *ileoce-cal valve*. This valve, or sphincter, opens and closes when chyme needs to pass through it, much as the pyloric sphincter does. In humans, the first part of the large intestine, the *ascending colon*, must transport the still-liquid chyme upward, against gravity. The ileocecal valve prevents fecal material from flowing back into the highly absorptive area of the ileum, yet still allows chyme to pass into the large intestine. When this valve malfunctions, we feel sick in many ways. If the valve remains open, waste is absorbed through the small intestine, and according to Joan Margaret, DC, contributes to *leaky gut* (personal communication, April 22, 2009). If the valve always stays closed, constipation is likely. Either way, IBS symptoms may result.

Getting the Most from What You Have

The final phase of the digestive process occurs in the large intestine, where we absorb the majority of water and dissolved minerals, and where waste material collects to be eliminated. If we are healthy, we harbor in the large intestine a large and varied population of beneficial bacteria (Reuter 2001) that digest soluble fiber, creating short-chain fatty acids that directly nourish the cells lining the large intestine. These bacteria also produce vitamin K and some B vitamins, and break down any remaining bile in the stool. More than four hundred species of bacteria live in our intestines, and the actual number of bacteria outnumbers the trillions of cells that make up our bodies. The semisolid waste (*feces*) consists of indigestible fiber (*cellulose*), bacteria (from one-third to one-half of fecal volume), and water. The large intestine removes water from the fecal material, and the final parts of the large intestine, the *sigmoid colon* and the *rectum*, collect it until the body eliminates it through the *anus*.

As we absorb the nutrients from the intestines into the bloodstream, they flow directly to the liver, where the blood is filtered, and nutrients are reassembled and either sent through the bloodstream to wherever they're needed or stored. The liver detoxifies harmful substances that have been absorbed from the intestine and, if they are water soluble, sends these now-harmless, neutralized compounds into the blood. The kidneys filter them into the urine and eliminate them. If the compounds are fat soluble, the liver puts them into the bile for the feces to eventually remove them. The liver also screens out pathogens and breaks them down for removal from the blood by way of the bile. Improperly neutralized toxins can cause many symptoms; still-toxic bile can irritate the intestines, leading to IBS symptoms (Joneja 2004).

When You Gotta Go

You've heard the saying, "You are what you eat," but more accurately, you are what you don't excrete. Ideally, having a bowel movement is effortless and efficient, and occurs one to three times a day, depending on how many meals you eat and their size. A healthy *transit time* (the time it takes for a meal to pass from mouth to anus) is eighteen to twenty-four hours. Defecation should take only a minute or less. The size of a normal stool is about eight to twelve inches long, and its shape is similar to a banana's. The consistency should be semisolid and uniform, and the color brown. The feces may float in the toilet briefly, and the smell shouldn't be extreme. You shouldn't see much residue on the toilet paper when you wipe, and should see no blood or mucus. If you chewed your food well, food particles aren't visible in the stool—no, not even corn.

Here in the Western world, the habit of sitting on a toilet makes having a bowel movement more difficult and can lead to chronic constipation, an IBS symptom. The majority of the world squats during defecation, and for good reason: the squatting position straightens the last part of the large intestine, improving the anal-rectal angle, allowing the feces to be pushed out easily and completely. Less straining means less potential to form hemorrhoids. In the squatting position, the thighs support the lower abdomen and promote proper action of the ileocecal valve. When we sit upright, the large intestine isn't as supported as it naturally is when we squat. How can you correct this? Elevate your feet on a small stool (no pun intended). You can buy an ergonomic squatting platform online or build one yourself. The Welles Step and the Lillipad are two such devices that fit around the modern toilet (see the resources for more information). You can even use a small trash can or a sturdy magazine rack for this purpose.

2

A Functional Problem with Many Causes

Eventually, poor digestion can result in the functional problem we call IBS. But why would digestion not function as efficiently or effortlessly as designed? What we put into our mouths directly affects the digestive system and can cause it to malfunction. Even our exposure to environmental toxins can directly contribute to IBS symptoms. All parts of the body are connected; problems in any area affect the whole.

EATING THE WRONG STUFF

One way to help your gut function optimally is to improve your overall health by laying a strong nutritional foundation. Humans have been around for about two hundred thousand years, and have survived and thrived by eating foods as nature provided. We were hunter-gatherers, eating many different animals and plants, depending on location and season. Around ten thousand years ago, we began adding dairy and then cereal grains to our diet. Humans learned—no doubt through trial and error—how to prepare these substances to make them edible and digestible. Cultural experiments with food production and processing continue, but we need to remember that it takes at least several generations to observe the full effects of changes we make. Anything less than a thousand years old is an experiment. We have been involved in an experiment of unprecedented proportions ever since the industrial revolution changed how food is produced.

Everything from how food is grown to how it's flavored has changed further in the last half century—and not always for the better. Petrochemical fertilizers, herbicides, pesticides, and preservatives are post–World War II inventions. Pesticide use has increased 3,300 percent since 1945, with only a 20 percent decline in crop losses (Crinnion 2000). Herbicides and pesticides applied to animal-feed crops may end up in commercial meat and dairy products. Our tissues absorb these poisons, damaging our digestive system and overall health.

Sugar, white rice, and white flour became widely available only 150 to 200 years ago. Refining of grains has changed: Flour production, once done by slow stone grinding, has become a highly mechanized milling process using metal rollers and extensive sieving. This refining process partially or entirely removes thirty-nine nutrients (Loiselle 1993). Processors are required by U.S. law to replace only five of these, and they do so with cheap synthetic versions.

The average American consumed 143 pounds of refined sweeteners (sugars and high-fructose corn syrup, or HFCS) in 2007, according to United States Department of Agriculture (USDA) food consumption data (USDA Sugar and Sweeteners Team 2008). This is the equivalent of more than three-quarters of a cup of sugar a day. Eating candy or drinking soft drinks is not required to consume this astounding amount. Sugar is hidden in almost all processed foods, including lunch meats and salad dressings. Each 12-ounce soda contains 12 to 16 teaspoons of sugar (or HFCS). Besides being empty calories, sugar creates imbalances of minerals, which are cofactors of vitamins and enzymes. Without adequate mineral balance, the vitamins you need to support you during stress are inactive (Lemann et al. 1970). (Sugar will be discussed further in chapter 5, but for a detailed description of sugar's negative effects, read *Lick the Sugar Habit*, by Nancy Appleton, published by Avery, 1996.)

Sugar can actually impair immunity, leading to overgrowth of pathogens in the digestive system, potentially resulting in IBS. According to doctors Michael Murray and Joseph Pizzorno (1998) in the *Encyclopedia of Natural Medicine*, white blood cells defend our health by eating a certain number of bacteria each hour, a number called the *lymphocytic index*. After consumption of the amount of refined carbohydrates in an evening meal on the standard American diet, about four ounces, the lymphocytic index decreases by 50 percent in the first hour and stays low for the next four to six hours. This depression of the immune system's functioning increases susceptibility to colds, flu, fungal infections, parasites, IBS, and even cancer.

Consuming these refined foods directly and negatively affects Americans' health and well-being in many ways, including causing digestive problems. For many years public health officials have urged us to increase fruit and vegetable consumption, with little change on our part. Refined foods can be physically and psychologically addictive, and their convenience crowds out healthy whole foods in many diets, with junk food now making up to 25 percent of the American diet (Block 2004). Statistics showing increases in all chronic diseases, including IBS, reveal a correlation when compared to consumption patterns. In the 1920s and 1930s, dentist Weston A. Price traveled around the world looking for populations that consumed traditional whole-food diets, and documented their general and dental health (Price 1945). He found that people who ate only whole, local foods, prepared traditionally, had excellent health and body structure. Dental cavities were rare until refined foods were consumed. After refined foods were introduced, subsequent generations had abnormalities of their dental arches, other bone deformities, narrowed facial structure, and the illnesses and chronic diseases considered common in Western civilization. Those who returned to their traditional diets regained all or most of their health, and their children born thereafter were healthy and strong.

EXPOSURE TO TOXINS

You can't expect your digestive system to function properly with imitation foods or chemically derived substances like those commonly found in the standard American diet. These substances can act as bowel irritants, especially when combined. We don't know all the health effects of the multitude of artificial substances in our food, beverages, and environment. A huge list of laboratory-created substances, some of which are food derived (such as MSG) or made from petroleum, is added to our foods (for example, preservatives such as BHA and BHT, food dyes, and flavorings). For instance, "white" wheat flour is bleached whiter with the chemical benzoyl peroxide, and has added oxidizers like potassium bromate, chlorine dioxide, and azodicarbonamide. You shouldn't need a chemistry degree to decide whether a food is good for you. Problems with food adulterations have been recognized since 1820, with Fredrick Accum's *A Treatise on Adulterations of Food and Culinary Poisons*. Food laws were enacted in the United States starting in the 1880s, culminating in the 1906 Pure Food and Drug Act. The public's desire for pure food has been around for a while, but it seems the legal definitions have changed along with the takeover of food manufacturing by fewer and larger corporations. Recent estimates indicate that 10 percent of the food the average American adult consumes consists of food additives, which is about 150 pounds of additives a person each year (Farrer 1987). Independent testing determined that 20 percent of these additives are carcinogenic in rats (Johnson 2002).

The Total Load Concept

Your digestive system's functioning depends on your overall health, especially the health of the liver. An overloaded liver can't neutralize toxins effectively, and the toxins in bile secreted from an overwhelmed liver can directly irritate the intestines, leading to IBS symptoms (Joneja 2004). We are living in a soup of man-made compounds; everything we breathe, smell, or spread on our skin or scalp can and does affect our health (Steinman and Wisner 1996). Everything we put on our skin is absorbed into the bloodstream (which is how analgesic creams and nicotine and estrogen patches work) and must be processed by the liver. Evidence is mounting to indicate that exposure to smog, plastics, and compounds in cosmetics and aerosol sprays causes problems (Ibid.). If we add up every instance of exposure to household chemicals, cosmetics, hidden chemicals we consume in our food, and environmental chemicals, we have a potent brew whose interactions in the body are totally unknown. While we can do little to immediately reduce chemical exposure outdoors, we can make many changes in our homes and diets that will help us avoid potentially harmful chemicals. Avoiding toxins allows the body to heal from many conditions, including IBS.

Imagine your body as a bucket with a spigot at the bottom. The spigot is your body's ability to neutralize (detoxify) and eliminate poisons (toxins). Every chemical you encounter contributes to filling up the bucket, which can be considered your total load (Bland and Benum 1997). Your exposure to chemicals determines how fast you fill your bucket. Your detoxification rate determines how open the spigot is and how easily it drains. If your rate of input equals that of emptying, your bucket is mostly empty and you aren't carrying around poisons. You have plenty of energy and no symptoms, and you feel good. If your input is very fast or contains something that can't pass through the spigot, the bucket will begin to fill up, and you may not feel as well while your body labors to get rid of the stuff in your bucket. If your spigot gets clogged or stops flowing, your bucket may fill up to the point of overflowing, causing many symptoms, including headaches, body aches, breathing difficulties, changes in blood flow, constipation or diarrhea, skin outbreaks or rashes, nerve tingling, and brain fog, or any combination of these. A toxin overload can contribute to any symptom or disease. If the liver can't completely neutralize the toxins you encounter, it may release them into the bile, which is secreted into the first part of the small intestine (duodenum). Some of these substances in the bile can irritate the small and large intestines, not only affecting their functioning, but also potentially damaging them, causing pain, swelling, and even inflammation. The presence of toxins in your body makes you feel tired and sick, and negatively affects bowel function (Nichols and Faass 1999). For more detailed information on how toxins can harm your digestion, read *Optimal Digestion*, edited by Dr. Trent Nichols and Nancy Faass (HarperCollins, 1999). (See Resources)

STRESS

Stress gets blamed for all kids of things, because it affects all aspects of how our bodies work, especially digestion. We undergo much more stress now than ever, being exposed to thousands of times as many stressors a day as people were just a hundred years ago (Stoll 1996).

Most people don't realize that stress comes in many forms and can have a wide-ranging effect on every bodily function, including memory, digestion, immunity, and sleep quality. Most people in our society think of stress as when traffic is backed up, you're late for an important appointment, your boss yells at you, or you are getting ready to meet your fiancé's entire family for the first time at Thanksgiving. These are mostly sociological and psychological stressors, but stressors can also be physical and environmental, or result from our own thoughts and emotions (see the following table). How we interpret our situation determines more about how our bodies react to stress than the actual situation; for example, losing your job can bring disabling anxiety, or you can look at it as an opportunity to find work that satisfies your soul.

In 1915 an American physiologist named Walter Cannon identified all organisms' reaction to real or perceived danger as "fright and fury" (Cannon 1915, 279), or, as we call it, the *fight-or-flight response*. In 1956 Dr. Hans Selye, a Canadian endocrinologist, redefined stress as "the nonspecifically induced changes within a biologic system" (Selye 1956, 54), and called any causative agent or demand a "stressor." No matter what is the source of the stress, the body responds to the change and tries to adapt to it.

Selye turned his own challenges into his life's work. His laboratory mice became ill and were dying from difficulties in handling them. Instead of ignoring what was happening to the mice, Selye studied it and discovered the many ways the body changes when the brain sounds an alarm. These changes, especially if the stress continues unabated, cause the body's repair and maintenance mechanisms to slow down or even stop. Digestion is impaired at all levels. Healing can slow down dramatically, because the immune system (much of it associated with digestion) is impaired, allowing opportunistic pathogens to proliferate, which can cause IBS symptoms (Nichols and Faass 1999), as I have also seen in my practice.

Type of Stress	Examples
Physical	Overwork, excess exercise, chemicals, junk food, accidents, surgery
Environmental	Pollution, noise, temperature extremes, electromagnetic fields, toxins
Biological	Illness, allergies, pain, chronic disease, hormone changes, aging, malnutrition
Sociological	Marriage, moving, work, daily hassles, caring for an ill loved one, loss, financial worries, birth, death
Psychological	Anger, fear, anxiety, frustration, negative thoughts, depression, sadness, grief

The digestive system requires considerable daily maintenance to stay healthy. When we are under stress, blood flow decreases to the digestive system and increases to the large muscles of the arms and legs (to fight or run), limbic brain, heart, and lungs. (Stress also reduces blood flow to the skin, reproductive system, immune system, and other organs not involved in immediate survival.) This means that when we are under stress, real or imagined, the oxygen and nutrients the digestive system uses for energy, and to replace and repair itself, are in short supply. If stress is ongoing, eventually the digestive system's organs will have difficulty providing nutrients to and moving waste from the body, resulting in a cycle of disease and degeneration. IBS is one of the symptoms of a digestive system's response to stress (Harvey 1989). Some people find that their thoughts and feelings trigger IBS symptoms such as diarrhea, spasms, constipation, or all three. Often, when an animal perceives danger, it will lighten its load and confuse its enemies by suddenly defecating before fleeing. For IBS sufferers, the gut's reaction to worry or anger may be the same.

Thankfully, by consistently practicing skilled relaxation, we can train the nervous system to remain calm. Quieting the nervous system by regularly practicing skilled relaxation reminds us we aren't walking at a cliff's edge, so our fight-or-flight response need not engage each time we stumble. Over time, this type of practice helps us reduce stored stress. Numerous methods are available, and different methods work for different people. As you grow and change, different types of skilled relaxation may work at different times in your life. For instance, transcendental meditation may work for you now, but you may find that a moving meditation, such as qigong, works better for you later in life. Numerous ways are available to get you into relaxation mode, such as: meditation; deep, slow diaphragmatic breathing; yoga; progressive muscle relaxation; mindfulness; repetitive exercise; imagery; receiving regular massage; and restful sleep. Additionally, tai chi, yoga, self-hypnosis, biofeedback, time management, and assertiveness training can also help you reduce stress and digest better (Davis, Eshelman, and McKay 1995). See chapter 5 for a simple relaxation technique.

OPPORTUNISTIC CRITTERS IN THE GUT: PATHOGENS AND PARASITES

We live in an environment with lots of other organisms, many of which, over time, we have evolved to have symbiotic relationships with. Bacteria that are friendly can help us digest food and actually create vitamins. These are often added to the diet in preparations called *probiotics*. Some bacteria that aren't so friendly are called pathogens or parasites. A *pathogen* is any organism that can contribute to disease or death. A *parasite* is an organism that feeds on and lives on, or in, another organism. These harmful organisms include some kinds of bacteria, fungi, yeast (candida), and microscopic animals, such as worms. According to nutrition expert Ann Louise Gittleman in her book *Guess What Came to Dinner*, many of us have encountered a variety of parasites in our lives, even if we have never traveled abroad (Gittleman 2001). Approximately 55 million Americans harbor parasites at some time in their lives, and we are host to more than 130 varieties (Ibid.). We can pick up these unwanted guests anywhere, by drinking contaminated water, while camping, or by eating improperly washed fruit or salad, or raw or undercooked meats, at home or in restaurants. Our pets are carriers, as are day care workers and food handlers. Even health care workers who don't wash their hands frequently or thoroughly enough can spread parasites. Municipal water systems frequently provide water that contains giardia, cryptosporidium, and other pathogens, which are resistant to chlorination.

Some symptoms of parasite infestation are quite similar to IBS symptoms: gas and bloating; overeating but still feeling hungry; alternating diarrhea and constipation; itchy anus, ears, and nose, especially at night; pain in the navel; forgetfulness; drooling while sleeping; and waking up in the middle of the night with a bellyache or racing thoughts. Symptoms are many, varied, and sometimes cyclic. Many people don't have distinctly digestive symptoms. These critters excrete toxins that can cause digestive and nondigestive symptoms, such as allergies, arthritis, asthma, chronic fatigue, and nerve disorders (Marx 1996). Many people become asymptomatic after initial exposure and write it off as food poisoning or "stomach flu."

Standard parasite treatments involve the use of pretty strong medicines and antibiotics, but overusing antibiotics can create "superbugs," pathogens that have adapted to become resistant to some of the strongest antibiotics. Unfortunately these critters are masters of disguise, with the ability to burrow into mucous membranes to keep from being swept away by digested food as it passes along the intestines. They can also migrate to other organs, such as the liver, lungs, heart, ovaries, and prostate (Ibid.), as well as attach to the intestinal lining. They can even coat themselves with our cells so our immune system won't recognize them as foreign. If you have IBS, get tested by a lab that specializes in parasites and seek holistic treatment from a practitioner experienced in parasitology (see the resources).

Using antibiotics can cause another problem, yeast overgrowth, also known as *candidiasis*. *Candida albicans* lives naturally in the large intestine, where sufficient amounts of good bacteria control its numbers. Antibiotics kill all bacteria, including the friendly ones, thus allowing candida growth to go unchecked. Add a diet high in sugar, sodas, and white flour products, and the candida are ready to party—a party that may leave you with a serious hangover (literally). Yeast plus sugar produce alcohol and many other toxic compounds. Candida is known to invade the intestinal walls and create *intestinal hyperpermeability*, also known as leaky gut. This and other pathogens expose our bloodstream to our digestive system's contents, potentially leading to food allergies and sensitivities—all of which may contribute to IBS.

IBS symptoms and leaky gut are often the result of exposure to contaminants. A common fungal contaminant in grains (deoxynivalenol) can increase intestinal permeability (Pinton et al. 2009). When foreign substances enter the bloodstream, the immune system goes into high gear. *Histamines* are released, causing swelling of the area to allow the immune-system cells to enter the tissues to do their work. White blood cells (WBCs) go to the area and engulf the invaders. If the WBCs are overwhelmed and can't eliminate the threat, stage two of the body's defense system swings into action: antibodies are produced that are specific to each invader. The antibody response protects us but can lead to food allergies and sensitivities.

EATING THE WRONG STUFF FOR YOU: FOOD ALLERGIES AND SENSITIVITIES

Even perfectly wholesome and whole foods can cause IBS or other digestive problems if you are even mildly allergic to or intolerant of that particular food or combination of foods (Gaby 1998). The body's production of antibodies (immumoglobulins) defines an allergy. Until recently the only antibodies easily measured, and thus recognized as allergy related, were the IgE antibodies, the ones that cause sudden reactions of itching, hives, swelling, and even asphyxiation and death. Scientists have now observed that there are subtle and delayed reactions that also involve antibodies. These IgA and IgG antibodies are released in an effort to protect the body from perceived threat in the mucous membranes and the gut. Many food allergies (IgA and IgG mediated) have subtle but cumulative symptoms that may show up days after the allergenic foods are eaten.

Food intolerances are even harder to identify, because there's no medical test for them. Food intolerance is defined as the inability to digest or metabolize a food or food group. Intolerances cause digestive symptoms and, sometimes, other symptoms, such as fatigue, brain fog, gas, and pain. Using a well-planned elimination diet, followed by carefully trying individual foods to determine if symptoms occur (provocative food testing), determines sensitivity and intolerance to various foods. To link symptoms to specific foods, you must keep meticulous notes during the provocative diet due to possibly delayed responses.

Thankfully, a blood test for IgA and IgG antibodies can now detect delayed food allergies. Though blood testing is faster than provocative food testing, it's expensive, and no test is 100 percent accurate or precise, but most tests can determine at least 94 percent of the foods you react to (Friel 2006; Miller 2007). The proof is that once you totally avoid your trigger foods for a time (some suggest four months, others twenty-four months), symptoms completely disappear. It's important to vary the menu every day to avoid frequent repetition of foods and to prevent production of new antibodies and development of other food sensitivities.

Common symptom-causing foods include wheat, dairy, eggs, soy, corn, fish, nuts, sugar, citrus, cocoa, and yeast.

HORMONE IMBALANCES

Women have IBS more often than men, and some women have more severe symptoms around the menstrual cycle. *Hormones* are chemical messengers made by glands and sent through the bloodstream to organs or other glands. The hormones actually attach to receptors on our cells, where they influence cells' actions. The stress hormone adrenaline (also known as epinephrine) is a good example. A sense of danger stimulates the pituitary gland (attached to the lower part of the brain) to secrete into the blood a hormone that quickly reaches the adrenal glands, which have receptors for it. The adrenals then secrete adrenaline, which goes through the blood to all parts of the body, signaling the body to react with a fight-or-flight response. All of this happens within seconds. After the cells receive and read these messages, the hormones are released from the cell wall, traveling back through the bloodstream until the liver quickly deactivates them.

Your liver is a busy organ, processing all the nutrients in the blood that come from the digestive system, neutralizing all the toxic materials in the blood, producing many proteins, and packaging cholesterol for distribution through the body. The liver also deactivates the hormones and plays an important role in regulating blood sugar. With all these tasks, it's no wonder the liver can become overwhelmed. Excess toxins are one challenge, but so is an overload of stress hormones, blood-sugar regulation, and other hormones (such as insulin and glucagon, and the sex hormones: estrogen, progesterone, and testosterone). During menopause the balance of sex hormones changes (dramatically in some women), adding to the burden both on the adrenals (since they take up the slack and make some sex hormones) and on the liver, to deactivate these hormones. These deactivated hormones are then excreted into the bile, which is eventually secreted into the small intestine after a meal or snack to help digest fats (see chapter 1). In the absence of adequate healthful bacteria (also known as probiotics) in the large intestine, the enzyme beta-glucuronidase can reactivate estrogen, which can then be reabsorbed back into the bloodstream from the large intestine creating a hormone imbalance (Nichols and Faass 1999). (If you are constipated, there's more time for this to happen.)

Hormone imbalances, birth control pills, and hormone replacement therapy are known to stimulate yeast growth, which contributes to leaky gut, food allergies, and IBS symptoms (Trowbridge and Walker 1986). Maintaining hormone balance can help reduce IBS symptoms dramatically. Avoiding meat and dairy products treated with hormones, avoiding pesticides and plastics (which act like hormones), getting adequate sleep and relaxation, and going outside and getting natural light are some good ways to maintain overall hormonal balance. Holistic health care practitioners use saliva tests for hormone levels to determine if you are in the normal ranges for your age and gender. Saliva tests identify the hormones that are bound to the tissues, not just those circulating in the blood, and therefore identify active hormones.

3

One Person's Food Is Another's Poison

To overcome IBS, it's important to identify any foods that contribute to your symptoms. There are two ways to find out what your body reacts to. One is practically free, but requires careful planning and record keeping; it's the elimination diet with provocative food testing and journal keeping. The other way is expensive ($350 to $500) but faster, and involves consulting a licensed health care professional to order a blood test for IgG and IgA antibodies. (See the resources to find laboratories that provide this service.) Though the blood tests (ELISA or RAST) are fairly accurate, no laboratory test is 100 percent accurate. Skin tests are even less accurate for food allergies (Friel 2006). When you have physical reactions to food allergens while on an elimination diet with provocative food testing, you can easily believe the results. This chapter will walk you step by step through the elimination diet.

THE ELIMINATION DIET

Here's how the elimination diet works: For at least one week, you eat only foods you don't regularly eat but know you aren't allergic to. Then, you'll add foods back into your diet one at a time, in their simplest form, carefully noting any reactions.

Choosing Foods

Your first step is to choose foods to eat during the first stage. If you know you are allergic to a food, avoid it, even if it's suggested as healthy or recommended for the elimination diet. Anyone can be allergic to anything! Foods least likely to produce an allergy include the following (the calories listed are a guide for adequate consumption):

Foods Least Likely to Produce Allergy			
Lamb	51 cal/oz.	Onions	11 cal/oz.
Fish (especially cod, haddock, mackerel, and trout)	30–50 cal/oz.	Parsnips	20 cal/oz.
Artichokes	15 cal/oz.	Peaches	11 cal/oz.
Beets and their greens	12 cal/oz.	Pears	16 cal/oz.
Carrots	10 cal/oz.	Rutabagas	11 cal/oz.
Celery	4 cal/oz.	Turnips and their greens	6 cal/oz.
Fennel bulbs	9 cal/oz.	Zucchini	4 cal/oz.
Green beans	10 cal/oz.	Any fresh vegetable or fruit you consume no more often than twice a week	

You can eat these foods in any amount and combination. If you regularly eat any of these foods more than twice a week, avoid it during the elimination phase of the diet. All food should be fresh, organic, and whole. Don't eat canned, frozen, dried, or other prepackaged foods, since cross-contamination often occurs in food processing. The immune system will detect even microscopic amounts of a food. Don't add spices or seasonings except for a dash of mineral salt or sea salt. Commercially refined salts contain dextrose (which is a sugar) calcium silicate, and aluminum silicate or ammonium citrate for dryness. You can bake, broil, or steam fish or lamb; and you can steam, bake, or boil vegetables. Don't eat fried foods. The only beverage you should drink is springwater or distilled water, since many people react to the chlorine and fluoride in treated water (Morris et al. 1992; Amira, Soufane, and Gharzouli 2005). Also, stop using any supplements and herbal remedies during this elimination phase.

Elimination Diet Sample Meals	
Breakfast	Ground lamb patty, steamed beets, beet greens, and zucchini
Snack	Celery and carrot sticks
Lunch	Lamb stew with green beans, onion, and parsnip
Snack	Steamed artichoke heart
Dinner	Baked fish, baked fennel and turnips, steamed carrots, and turnip greens
Snack	Fresh or poached pear

How Much Should I Eat on the Elimination Diet?

How much you eat on the elimination diet isn't as important as how you eat. Be mindful. Eat slowly and chew thoroughly. Eat until you are satisfied or until your stomach feels three-quarters full. Eat three meals, and include snacks if you feel hungry. Just make sure all meals and snacks consist of only the allowed foods.

How Will I Feel on the Elimination Diet?

Withdrawal symptoms often occur during the elimination diet. You are no longer receiving the druglike endorphin boost you get from consuming allergenic foods (Brostoff and Gamlin 2000). Withdrawal symptoms can include headache, joint pain, muscle aches, fatigue, and other flu-like symptoms. Most, if not all, symptoms should clear by the end of the fourth day, and you can expect increased energy by day six (Clarke et al. 1996). After completely avoiding their problem foods, some people find that they feel better than they have in years.

Another way to heal the intestines is a modified version of the elimination diet, as described by Elaine Gottschall (1994) in *Breaking the Vicious Cycle*. Eat only homemade chicken-vegetable soup morning, noon, and night for three weeks for the following reasons:

- You can control all of the ingredients in a homemade-from-scratch soup, thereby avoiding any potential allergens.

- The compounds in homemade bone broth are particularly soothing to the digestive tract and important for healing leaky gut (Siebecker 2005).

- Soups offer nutrients in liquid form, making them easy to digest and absorb.

- Soups are simple to prepare, and can be made in large batches and frozen for convenience.

- Chicken soup is a traditional comfort food in many cultures.

Three weeks may seem like a long time to consume only soup for all meals. To avoid becoming bored with this limited diet, vary somewhat the combinations of vegetables used in the soup, for instance, chicken-carrot soup, chicken-onion-celery soup, chicken-zucchini soup, and so on. In the next stage, you can add more foods, increasing your menu variety.

Provocative Food Testing

After you've been on the elimination diet until your symptoms have cleared, around three weeks for most people (Gottschall 1994), you can begin provocative food testing by adding whole, unrefined foods back into your diet, one every third day (seventy-two hours), to see if allergy symptoms return. I suggest beginning by adding foods you suspect aren't problematic, to widen your dietary choices and extend your symptom-free period, allowing the gut to heal. Eat each test food in its purest state (such as fluid milk instead of cheese, or raw tomato instead of salsa). Consume just one serving of the food, preferably by itself. Notice and record how you feel. After about an hour, consume foods on your elimination diet. Wait three days (seventy-two hours) before adding another provocative food, even if you don't feel any symptoms immediately on the first or second day. Once a food proves not to cause symptoms, you can add it to your diet, ideally on a four-day rotation schedule, which I'll describe next. A food-symptom journal is essential at this point to identify all forms of allergy symptoms, including energy and mood disorders, not just bowel symptoms (see the form in the next section). Adding potentially allergenic foods (provocative food testing) takes time and careful attention so you can determine how you feel. If you react to a food, wait until the symptoms go away. Only then can you test another food and monitor your reactions.

Be aware that your reaction to a problem food may be quite uncomfortable. After your body clears the residues of any food it considers toxic, it has the energy to react to the reintroduced food with full force. Feeling a physical or emotional reaction to a food, to the extent you can directly associate it with that food, motivates you to completely avoid that food in the future, making it easier to commit to long-lasting dietary changes.

The Rotation Diet

Once provocative food testing proves a food doesn't cause symptoms, you can add it to your diet, but not every day. After you determine which foods don't cause symptoms, a four-day (or longer) rotation diet is necessary to prevent you from developing new allergic reactions to those foods. It takes approximately four days for the immune system to begin producing antibodies to an invader. Only an invasion that's severe or lasts for at least this period is considered enough of a threat to warrant antibody production. If you consume a food only once every four days, the body doesn't feel the need to expend the energy required to protect you from the random or infrequent assault.

If all this sounds too complicated, don't worry. Examples of an elimination diet plan and rotation plan are outlined in chapter 7. Uncovering your trigger foods is a big relief, compared to the frustration of not knowing what's causing your symptoms. Once you know what to avoid and what to eat, the real healing can begin.

KEEPING A FOOD-SYMPTOM JOURNAL

Tracking your diet and symptoms is essential to understanding what triggers your IBS symptoms. Using a diary or journal is a necessary tool to find what works for you. Having the information in writing keeps you from forgetting the details of what food you ate or the reactions it caused, which can occur up to three days later. Use a scoring system to make record keeping fast and easy. When you take time to review a few weeks of your food diary, you can usually identify patterns of foods, activities, stress, and symptoms, even if the patterns aren't initially discernible. You may want to seek help from a nutritionist, because it's difficult to be as objective as others about your own situation. Anyone can be allergic or sensitive to anything. You may find you aren't sensitive to a food by itself, but have symptoms when you combine it with another food. Or you may find you are sensitive to a food only when under stress, or when you are also exposed to an inhalant allergen, such as seasonal pollen or mold. The combinations of foods, stressors, and activity or exercise can amplify reactions, resulting in bowel symptoms. Here's a template you can photocopy to help you record your foods and symptoms.

DAILY FOOD-SYMPTOM JOURNAL

Date	Food Eaten (and Approximate Amount)	Activity or Exercise	Mood 1–10	Stress Level 1–10	Symptoms
Time: Breakfast					
Time: Snack					
Time: Lunch					
Time: Snack					
Time: Dinner					
Time: Snack					

Symptom key: D = diarrhea, C = constipation, P = pain, G = gas, B = bloating, O = other

■ Case Study: Daniel

Here's the story of a health-conscious young man who was able to heal very quickly and completely, because he was meticulous with his food diary and rotation diet. Daniel, aged twenty-six, had extreme fatigue and abdominal pain after all meals, and was experiencing weight loss. His stools varied from loose to soft, with some pain relief after evacuation. The stool test from his doctor was negative for parasites, and an endoscopy showed nothing unusual. He was handed the IBS diagnosis and told nothing could be done. His weight loss continued. Then a stool test from a specialized lab (see the resources) revealed antibodies to tapeworm and roundworm. After treatment with an appropriate prescription drug, he passed many worm segments and gradually began feeling better. After three weeks on a whole-food elimination diet, during which his symptoms continued to abate, he adopted a rotation diet. With careful record keeping, he was able to identify and avoid trigger foods. He has regained his lost weight and, after one year, no longer has any IBS symptoms. His health continues to improve on a rotation diet of whole foods tailored to his digestive needs.

The following chart shows Daniel's progress based on his responses to a health-appraisal questionnaire assessing symptoms at intake and after sixteen months on his treatment plan.

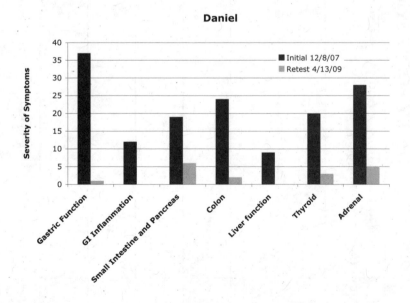

Figure 3.1   Daniel's Progress

4

Back to the Basics

It's hard to talk about nutritional support for any health condition without first describing particular food groups. Thousands of years ago, all food was organic by default. Food processing consisted of simple cooking, grinding, fermenting, or drying. Salt, local spices, and herbs were the only food additives. We got everything we needed from the food because it was whole, unadulterated, and fresh. If we go back to eating only whole, fresh, organic local foods, our diet will provide the nutrition we need to thrive. Unfortunately, today this isn't so easy without an understanding of basic nutrition to guide our food selections. Once we know what nutrients the foods contain, we can choose our meals more wisely to heal IBS.

THE BUILDING BLOCKS OF A HEALTHY BODY

You know we all need food to survive, but you may not know you need specific nutrients, not just calories, for your body to function efficiently. Only whole foods can provide you with the proper combination of nutrients you need. No synthetic vitamin or mineral supplement can substitute for a whole food. Under certain circumstances, you can add specific combinations of vitamin and mineral complexes to a healthy diet as supplements, but whole foods must be the foundation of the healing process.

You need several ounces of some nutrients a day, such as protein, fats, and carbohydrates—known as macronutrients. Other nutrients, including vitamins and minerals, antioxidants, fiber, and fluids—which you need in much smaller amounts—conveniently occur in whole food in the exact ratios your body requires. Because the digestive system is the first part of your body to encounter the foods you eat, it's important to eat foods in as simple a form as possible, unrefined and unadulterated. Your digestion is well adapted to whole foods and the abundance of nutrients naturally therein. Is it any wonder that when you eat foods that are deficient in one or more nutrients, or that contain additives, your digestive system (and the rest of your body) may not function optimally?

Proteins

Essential for growth and repair, proteins are the building blocks of all parts of your body. Everything from the skin, hair, nails, brain, nerves, liver, heart, and small intestine to immunity requires adequate protein. Your digestive system both requires and provides protein each day. Made up of amino acids, proteins are in all whole and unprocessed foods in at least small amounts. Quantity and proportion of amino acids vary for each food, so it's essential to eat a wide variety of foods. Good vegetable sources of protein are combinations of legumes (beans and peas), nuts and seeds, grains, mushrooms, microalgae, and seaweeds.

Depending on your size and activity level, to heal from any illness you need about three to five ounces of protein-rich foods two to three times a day. A three-ounce serving of lean beef sirloin contains 25 grams of protein. A piece of meat or fish the size of your palm or a deck of cards is considered an appropriate serving size of protein-rich foods. Meat, poultry, dairy, eggs, and fish are the most concentrated sources of protein, but when consumed without balancing with vegetables (as in the standard American diet), they tend to acidify tissues, increasing your need for calcium, magnesium, and other alkalinizing minerals due to protein's high concentration of phosphorous (Frassetto et al. 2001). Unless organically and naturally raised, meat and dairy products contain numerous hormones, antibiotics, and toxic chemicals.

Fats and Oils

Fats and oils are essential for energy, growth, and insulation. You need fats to build your body's cell walls, brain cells, and hormones, to insulate nerves, and to carry the fat-soluble vitamins (A, D, E, and K). The right kinds of fats in the correct ratios help the entire body, including the digestive, nervous, and immune systems. Without fats your cells dry out and your membranes are less flexible.

In the late 1970s, scientists found that some fats are absolutely necessary for health, and unlike saturated fats, our bodies can't make them. You must get these fats from your diet, which is why they're called *essential fatty acids* (*EFAs*). There are two types of EFAs: omega-3 and omega-6. Both are required in your diet for you to regain and maintain health. Good-quality omega-6 fat sources are: fresh, raw nuts and seeds; whole grains; and beans. Omega-3 fat sources are: flaxseeds; hemp, chia, and pumpkin seeds; walnuts; and cold-water ocean fish, such as sardines, salmon, tuna, and black cod. A healthy ratio of omega-6 to omega-3 fatty acids is between 3 to 1 and 1 to 1. The average American consumes twenty times as much omega-6 as omega-3 fats (a ratio of 20 to 1) (Rudin and Felix 1996). This imbalance can contribute to inflammation and pain in any part of the body, including the gut, leading to IBS symptoms. Function depends on form, and creating form requires all nutrients. Fatty acids are incorporated into the lipid bilayer of all membranes. Proper functioning of membranes depends on the correct ratio of these fatty acids (and all nutrients and enzymes) (Enig 2000). Those with IBS may need to consume foods rich in omega-3 fatty acids, such as fatty fish, or take fish oil supplements, preferably as high-vitamin cod-liver oil, which includes the fat-soluble vitamins.

Most packaged foods in supermarkets contain many overprocessed and poor-quality fats. To avoid illness and efficiently rebuild intestinal health, it's important to totally avoid hydrogenated and partially hydrogenated oils, such as margarines, shortenings, and oils heated above 320 degrees Fahrenheit (all fried foods). Frying foods always damages and oxidizes fats. Read all ingredient labels carefully to avoid hydrogenated, partially hydrogenated, and refined vegetable oils. Partially hydrogenated fats often contain trans-fatty acids that contribute to disease and prevent healing. Even when the nutrition facts label lists 0 grams of trans fats, manufacturers are allowed to include 0.5 grams or less *per serving*. The manufacturer determines the serving size, which may be smaller than is realistic. Thus when you eat what seems like a serving, you may get more trans fats than the government considers safe. Some USDA researchers indicate there's no safe level of trans fats in the diet (Ibid.).

Which fats are good to use? Use only organic, unrefined oils, such as extra-virgin olive, cold-pressed flaxseed, or hemp oil for salad dressings. Never cook with flaxseed oil since it's quite sensitive to heat, and store it in the freezer to prevent rancidity longer; it will remain liquid. Organic butter or ghee (clarified butter) is much healthier and better tasting than any margarine for cooking and baking. But both contain at least some milk protein, so if you are sensitive to dairy, you may need to avoid butter and ghee. Unrefined coconut and palm oils have been used for centuries in many recipes calling for butter or margarine, and they don't cause heart disease, as was once thought (Simopoulos 2002). Use these naturally saturated fats to sauté or stir-fry, because they are unlikely to oxidize and become rancid. You can use coconut or palm oil for baking instead of shortening.

Carbohydrates

The body uses *carbohydrates* (sugars and starches) for energy. All carbohydrates and fiber originate from plants, and are a major source of vitamins and minerals if unrefined, especially if grown organically (Benbrook et al. 2008). Plants also provide as-yet-unidentified compounds that are necessary for health. Whole grains, beans, and vegetables are all excellent sources of unrefined complex carbohydrates. Whole grains are most digestible and nutritious if soaked, sprouted, or fermented before being eaten (Fallon and Enig 1999). Examples of unrefined grains are whole wheat, whole rye, hulled (not pearled) barley, oats, brown rice, millet, buckwheat, amaranth, quinoa (pronounced "keen-wa"), and whole cornmeal. Fruits such as berries, apples, pears, peaches, citrus, and melons are all excellent sources of unrefined carbohydrates. So are vegetables such as asparagus, onions, garlic, leeks, carrots, beets, all kinds of squash, spinach, chard, parsley, basil, cilantro, all leafy greens, and cruciferous vegetables, such as broccoli, cauliflower, cabbage, Brussels sprouts, kale, collards, radish, and mustard greens.

Sugar, fruit juice, white rice, white-flour baked products such as white bread, crackers, and white pasta, peeled potatoes, and other processed foods are some examples of refined carbohydrates. A vegetable's peel contains a considerable amount of its fiber, vitamins, and minerals (Davis 1970). Refined grains offer little more than empty calories due to the removal of nutrients (Ibid.). Enrichment of refined grains is woefully inadequate to regain or maintain health. Eating refined foods actually depletes the body of the vitamins and minerals necessary to use the food, leaving you wanting more (DeCava 2006).

Though a good source of vitamins, antioxidants, bioflavonoids, and fiber, fruit can elevate blood sugar in sensitive individuals. Juice is a refined food because the fiber has been removed, and if bottled or canned, it's usually preserved with chemicals and pasteurized, which destroys enzymes and some vitamins. When we eat a piece of fruit, as opposed to just the juice, the fiber that's present in whole fruit helps slow the release of carbohydrates as sugar into the bloodstream. This slower increase in blood sugar gives us the time to use the sugar for energy. If you don't have candidiasis (or other sugar-loving parasites) and don't have blood-sugar problems, enjoy one or two servings of fresh fruit a day. Eating large amounts of sweets, dried fruit, and even "naturally sweetened" health foods can cause IBS symptoms, just as refined sugar does. You may need to limit dried fruit, because it's a very concentrated sugar source that can feed bad bacteria, yeast, or both (causing IBS symptoms), and it's easy to eat too much of it.

What About Fiber?

Though humans can't digest fiber, we need it to regulate the bowels. Many carbohydrate-rich whole foods contain considerable fiber. Fiber absorbs and holds onto water, which makes the stool soft and moist, and easy to pass. We also need fiber to stabilize blood-sugar levels and even to help lower blood-cholesterol levels. (Fiber binds with cholesterol, and if you have one to three daily bowel movements, there's not enough time for the cholesterol to be reabsorbed back into the bloodstream to increase serum-cholesterol levels. Thus a high serum-cholesterol level may be a sign of a poorly functioning bowel and potential IBS.) Due to the fiber, whole complex carbohydrates help you feel full sooner, with fewer calories, and sustain you longer than refined carbohydrates.

Fiber is one of the most confusing topics for IBS sufferers. Everyone's different as far as the kind of fiber needed, how much, and when. According to the USDA's recommended dietary allowance, you need a minimum of approximately 30 grams of fiber each day to stay healthy (Cordain et al. 2005). The average American consumes only about half the recommended fiber. Whole-food, plant-based diets provide 30 to 50 grams of fiber a day, and traditional native diets provided even more (Ibid.). However, fiber consumption during a spell of painful IBS symptoms isn't always recommended. Fiber consumed without adequate water can make bricks! Suddenly adding large amounts of fiber to the diet can cause considerable gas and even diarrhea. Some kinds of fiber can irritate the intestines, depending on the source. If you have difficulty digesting whole grains or have more IBS symptoms when eating them, try starchy vegetables such as carrots, beets, winter squash, and yams instead of grains, to provide more-digestible carbohydrates that still contain the necessary fiber.

What's the difference between soluble and insoluble fiber? Fiber from whole foods is a mix of two kinds of fiber, soluble and insoluble, and you need both. *Soluble fiber* (also known as *mucilage*) is the slippery, gooey fiber that dissolves in water, and examples are pectin and inulin. Soluble fiber is in all vegetables and fruits and is a beneficial food for your healthful intestinal bacteria. After the bacteria consume the soluble fiber, they produce short-chain fatty acids (SCFAs) that are absorbed by the cells lining the large intestine. SCFAs are an energy source for our intestinal cells, and well-fed intestinal cells can function more easily and reduce IBS symptoms.

Unfortunately, if present in the colon, some harmful bacteria also feast on soluble fiber, creating painful by-products. One type of these bacteria is *klebsiella*, often found in hospital and clinical settings. If you have klebsiella and consume foods or supplements containing lots of soluble fiber, your IBS symptoms may increase dramatically. A stool test from a specialized laboratory can detect a klebsiella infection (see the resources).

Insoluble fiber, also known as *roughage*, is the kind of fiber most people associate with laxatives. It's the indigestible part of plants that doesn't dissolve in water. The bran of whole grains, such as wheat bran, is almost exclusively insoluble fiber. Other examples are vegetable and fruit skins, nuts, and seeds. You need insoluble fiber, but if it comes from foods you are sensitive to, you'll need other sources. If diarrhea is one of your IBS symptoms, avoid fiber supplements and, instead, eat plenty of fresh vegetables and fruits (which contain both kinds of fiber). If you have celiac disease or are wheat sensitive, wheat bran is not for you.

Both kinds of fiber absorb considerable water and, thus, swell to many times their original volume. Because fiber holds onto water, it creates the perfect volume and consistency to allow easy and complete passage of the stool along the large intestine. The large intestine can feel that there's a stool to move, so the muscle contractions of peristalsis occur. As it passes through the intestine, fiber gently cleans and stimulates the intestinal walls. Fiber also helps you eliminate cholesterol and steroid hormones present in the bile and secreted into the intestine. The healthful bacteria help break down caustic bile acids, preventing them from irritating the intestinal cells. Since fiber is food for your healthful bacteria, include it in your IBS diet, but obtain it primarily from foods, not supplements. Experiment with your consumption of high-fiber foods such as cooked leafy greens, artichoke, cucumber, broccoli, green beans, snow peas, mushrooms, leeks, and seaweed, and keep a diet-symptom diary. Everyone's different. If you notice that adding a food aggravates your IBS symptoms, consider avoiding it completely. Though high in fiber, grains and beans can irritate the large intestine, so replace them with fresh vegetables if necessary.

Micronutrients

Though micronutrients are essential, you need only very small amounts. They occur naturally and in perfect ratios in fresh, whole organic foods. Processing, heat, time, and oxygen can deplete micronutrients in foods, which is why it's important to choose in-season, unprocessed foods to optimize your micronutrient intake. There are likely many micronutrients yet to be discovered, and the only guaranteed source of these critical components of health is fresh, whole foods.

VITAMINS

Vitamins are essential to life, and we must get them from what we eat. Many studies have shown that the natural vitamins in whole foods have more health benefits than synthetic vitamin molecules or vitamins that have been separated from the foods in which they naturally exist (DeCava 2006). Every cell of your body needs every nutrient at all times. You need every vitamin and mineral in its naturally existing proportion in a wide variety of whole foods. Biochemical individuality means that everyone doesn't have exactly the same needs all the time. You require more vitamins and minerals during periods of growth, pregnancy, lactation, recovery from injury, illness, or stress. Vitamins act as cofactors in the work of the body, and are essential catalysts to all the body's actions, including digestion and healing IBS. Since IBS can interfere with absorption of some nutrients, it's important to supply all nutrients abundantly, which you can do only by eating a wide variety of fresh, whole foods, emphasizing the most nutrient-dense foods possible. The following table identifies the richest sources of the many vitamins needed for healing.

VITAMINS NEEDED FOR HEALING

Vitamins	Best Sources	Functions
A (retinol, ß-carotene) ☆	Organic liver, fish, eggs and dairy from pasture-raised animals, poultry and meat, dark-green and deep-orange vegetables and fruit	Facilitates growth and repair of cell and mucous membranes; helps form bones and teeth; enhances vision and immunity
B-1 (Thiamin) ⌀	Organic liver, yeast, nuts, meat, fish, wheat germ, whole grains, beans, peas	Nerve function, muscle tone, carbohydrate metabolism
B2 (riboflavin) ⌀☆	Meat, dairy, yeast, green leafy vegetables, whole grains, beans, nuts	Helps immunity, regulates metabolism, helps brain functioning, facilitates B6 metabolism
B3 (niacin)	Fish, meat, dairy, eggs, beans, whole grains, nuts	Metabolizes proteins, carbohydrates, and fats, helps blood circulation

Vitamins	Best Sources	Functions
B5 (pantothenic acid)	Organ meats, meats, whole grains, legumes	Metabolizes vitamins, carbohydrates, and fats for energy, supports adrenals
B6 (pyridoxine) ✍☆	Dairy, fish, meat, sprouted grains, raw wheat germ, raw nuts, yeast	Helps brain functioning, prevents PMS, helps carpal tunnel syndrome, reduces cholesterol
B12 (cobalamin) ✍☆	Organ meats, eggs, dairy, meat, fish, fortified nutritional yeast	Increases mental agility and coordination; necessary for nerve functioning
Biotin	Egg yolks, dark-green vegetables, whole grains, healthful intestinal bacteria	Metabolizes proteins, fats, and carbohydrates; helps other B vitamins
Folic acid ✍☆	Organ meats, nutritional yeast, leafy vegetables, dried beans, whole grains	Forms red blood cells, metabolizes protein, assists growth and nerve functioning
C complex ✍	Citrus fruit, fresh fruit, and vegetables	Is an antioxidant; enhances immunity, repairs tissues, forms collagen, detoxifies, prevents bruises
D (cholecalciferol) ✍☆	Cod-liver oil (the high-vitamin type), direct sunshine on skin oils (sans sunscreen*), pasture-raised meat and dairy, fish	Forms bones and teeth, metabolizes calcium, enhances immunity, balances mood, facilitates intestinal health
E (tocopherols)	Wheat germ, seeds, nuts, vegetable oils (unrefined), dark-green leafy vegetables, whole grains, sweet potatoes	Is an antioxidant; protects cell membranes, nerves, red blood cells, hormones, and vitamin A

K (phylloquinone)	Green leafy vegetables, whole grains, fruit, eggs, healthful intestinal bacteria, fermented soybeans, sprouts	Forms blood clots, repairs bones, prevents osteoporosis
Lecithin	Egg yolk, liver, whole grains, beans, unrefined oil	Balances cholesterol, helps brain and nerve functioning

⊘Sensitive to heat; fresh or raw is best

☆Light sensitive

*Overexposure to sunlight burns the skin, but we need moderate sun exposure to make vitamin D. The amount of sun needed depends on season, latitude, smog, and skin color. Visit www.vitamindcouncil.org for more information on vitamin D.

MINERALS

Without the complete variety and proportions of minerals found in whole foods, we couldn't sustain life. Minerals are needed in every bodily function, not just to provide hardness to our bones. Minerals are cofactors with vitamins to: heal and repair gut tissue; move our muscles, such as in peristalsis; create the digestive enzymes that allow us to digest our food; supply our immune system with the ability to defend us from pathogens; and help us detoxify. We know of twenty minerals the body requires in amounts from grams to micrograms. (One gram is the weight of a paper clip, and one microgram is one millionth of a gram.) The result of inadequate amounts of any mineral is poor digestive function or other signs of ill health. Stress increases elimination of minerals via the urine (Selye 1956). Refined carbohydrates, in general, and sugar, specifically, deplete the body of the minerals needed for good intestinal health. Because each cell requires minerals and vitamins to metabolize glucose (sugar) to produce energy, if these minerals aren't provided by the foods that supply the glucose (as they aren't with sugar and refined carbohydrates), the cell must borrow the required nutrients from its stores. Continued borrowing leads to increased deficit, which manifests in your body as fatigue, dysfunction, and finally illness (Yudkin 1972). Without adequate amounts of the health-supporting minerals you need, your body may absorb toxic minerals, also known as *heavy metals*. Some examples of heavy metals are aluminum, arsenic, cadmium, lead, and mercury. They disrupt normal enzyme functions and interfere with healing, nerve conduction, muscle movement (potentially causing chronic constipation), and immune system defenses (Quig 1998).

MINERALS NEEDED FOR HEALING

Minerals	Best Sources	Functions
Calcium	Fish with bones (sardines, canned salmon), dairy,* seaweeds, green leafy vegetables, nuts, seeds	Builds bones and teeth, calms nerves, soothes pain, contracts muscles, helps with blood clotting
Magnesium	Dark-green leafy vegetables and seaweeds, wheat germ, whole grains, beans, nuts, seeds	Relaxes muscles, helps calcium and potassium metabolism and B-complex utilization, activates enzymes
Sodium	Sea salt, seaweeds, seafood, celery, green leafy vegetables	Balances potassium, helps with adrenal function, needed during extreme heat or stress
Potassium	Vegetables, fruits, seaweeds, dairy, beans, whole grains, seeds	Balances fluid, controls nerve and muscle activity
Iron	Organic liver, fish, eggs, green leafy vegetables, seaweeds, dried fruits, blackstrap molasses	Forms hemoglobin in blood and myoglobin in muscles, supplies oxygen to cells
Zinc	Oysters, seafood, organic liver, seaweeds, pumpkin seeds, whole grains, beans, yeast, eggs from pasture-raised hens	Facilitates wound healing and immunity, produces stomach acid, facilitates reproductive health, enzyme metabolism, appetite, and sense of smell and taste
Iodine	Seafood, seaweeds, dairy, egg yolk, iodized salt	Supports thyroid, immunity, and detoxification, supports antioxidants, prevents cysts
Chromium	Organ meats, whole grains, nutritional yeast, seaweeds	Regulates energy, metabolizes glucose, helps B-complex functioning

Minerals	Best Sources	Functions
Copper [*]	Beans, nuts, dried fruit, seaweeds, fish	Facilitates bone growth and blood formation, works with vitamin C to form elastin protein
Manganese [*]	Seaweeds, whole grains, fruits, green leafy vegetables, nuts, seeds	Activates enzymes, metabolizes carbohydrates and fats, balances hormones, assists skeletal development and coordination
Selenium [*]	Seaweed, fish, whole grains, tree nuts, nutritional yeast	Is an antioxidant, supports immunity, protects against radiation and pollution
Sulfur	Eggs, garlic, onions, leeks, cruciferous vegetables, alfalfa sprouts, beans	Metabolizes protein and amino acid, supports immunity, detoxifies

[*] These minerals are frequently deficient in nonorganic sources (Benbrook et al. 2008).

*The minerals are much more available to the body when the enzymes in the milk are present, and pasteurization destroys enzymes (Schmid 2009; Pottenger 1938; Crewe 1929). Please check with your health care provider to see if certified raw dairy products are a safe option for you.

Using the Eating4Health Model

The Eating4Health model is a regenerative food system to help you organize and plan meals and menus. Created by Edward Bauman, Ph.D., and used extensively by holistic nutrition consultants, the model shows a plateful of possibilities for healthy food and beverage choices (Bauman 2008). It emphasizes seasonal, organic, unrefined, and local foods (what I call SOUL foods). If you have digestive problems or IBS, emphasize leafy and crunchy vegetables; good-quality whole-food proteins with their naturally accompanying fats; *booster foods* that speed up metabolism, such as spices and seaweed; and natural beverages. You may need to limit or eliminate some unrefined starches and fruits to avoid IBS symptoms. This model serves as a guide to choosing a wide variety of whole foods.

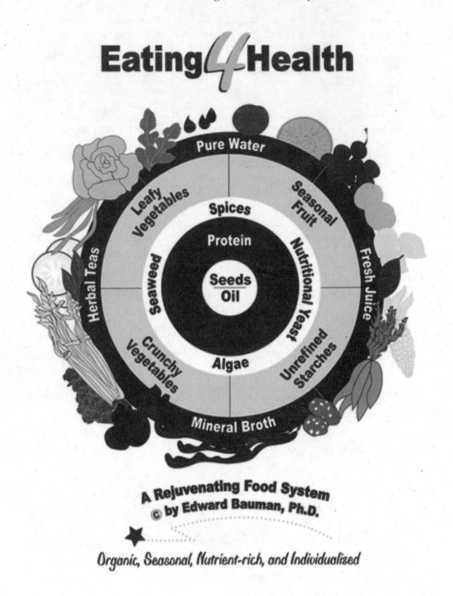

Figure 4.1   Eating4Health

Eating4Health Foods and Serving Sizes

	Seeds and Oils	Protein	Leafy Vegetables	Crunchy Vegetables	Unrefined Starches	Seasonal Fruit	Booster Foods
Daily Servings	2–3	2–4	1–3	1–3	2–4	2–4	2–4
Serving Size	1 tbs. oil 2 tbs. seeds	3 oz. animal 6 oz. vegetable	1 cup	1/2 cup	1/2 cup root vegetable, grains, bread	1/2 cup or 1 med. piece	1 tsp.–1 tbs.
Examples	flax sunflower sesame chia pumpkin	poultry fish eggs milk beans (including lentils) meat	salad mix kale chard cabbage parsley cilantro spinach	broccoli string beans onion celery cucumber	yam winter squash corn millet brown rice	berries apple pear grapes fig citrus	spices yeast algae seaweed

©2008 Ed Bauman, Ph.D, www.baumancollege.org

CHAPTER 5

What You Can Do to Help Your Gut

Change is hard, but the hardest thing to change is your mind. Once you do that, it's much easier to adjust your behavior to accomplish your goals. If you do the same things you've always done, you'll get the same results you've always had. Your distressing IBS symptoms are undoubtedly enough to convince you that some sort of change is necessary.

You can change three things to overcome IBS: how you react to your environment, how much you move your body, and what you put into it. You may wonder, "What should I do first?" The answer is whatever you *can* do. Start now making the easiest changes for you, and watch your overall quality of life improve.

STRESS AND IBS

Start by taking a slow, deep breath; then another and another. Repeat for five to twenty minutes twice a day. Regular relaxation is an often-ignored activity you can do (at no cost) to help your bowel begin functioning properly again. Many good books are available that describe the numerous ways to increase the relaxation response. (See "Relaxation Aids and Information" in the resources.)

For your body to heal and recover from IBS, you must first allow it the time and energy to do so, which is best achieved with eight or more hours of sound, restful sleep each night and daily practice of any form of effective skilled relaxation, such as those described in *The Relaxation and Stress Reduction Workbook*. These methods include breathing techniques, meditation, visualization, biofeedback, self-hypnosis, yoga, tai chi, and qigong. Do whatever works best for you to achieve deep relaxation.

The Importance of Skilled Relaxation

Skilled relaxation differs from just reading a book or zoning out in front of the television. Many of us spend too much time disconnected from ourselves but connected to our electronic devices, rushing, working, and taking care of others. You may have to give yourself the gift, the permission, to "do nothing" in the sense of just being present in your own body, feeling and listening to your breath.

Your brain and the rest of your nervous system constantly strike a balance between the *parasympathetic* and *sympathetic nervous systems*, which are two sides of the same coin. Ideally you need to spend the majority of your time in a calm and relaxed state (parasympathetic mode) to do all the maintenance and repair the body requires, but you still need to be able to quickly respond to any challenge, good or bad, that confronts you (sympathetic mode). When you intentionally do any form of skilled relaxation, you can again engage the parasympathetic nervous system and receive all of its benefits.

When you are stimulated or frightened, or under any form of stress, your body responds with physical changes that affect how you feel in both the short and long terms. Any feeling of danger, real or imagined, activates the sympathetic nervous system, and you respond directly to your environment with action. When you are nervous, your breathing becomes faster but shallower. You may even feel that you aren't getting enough air, so you sigh and yawn to get more oxygen to your brain. One of the most common symptoms of sympathetic nervous system dominance (stress) is cold hands and feet. (See chapter 2 for more information on the relationship between stress and IBS.)

When we are calm and relaxed, our parasympathetic nervous system dominates: Our hands and feet are warm and dry (even when the weather isn't). Breathing is regular and deep. Our blood flow is balanced and nourishes our internal organs. We can more easily digest food, resist pathogens, and heal any injury. IBS symptoms recede.

The Power of the Breath

The breath is the symbol and definition of life in many cultures and languages. Breathing deeply and slowly profoundly affects the levels of oxygen that get to the brain and all organs. Oxygen helps us provide healing energy to every cell, including intestinal cells. Deep breathing can help relieve constipation and reduce IBS abdominal pain. It also aids the liver's detoxification of the blood and helps carry nutrients to each cell. When you breathe deeply into your belly, the layer of muscles between the lungs and abdomen, known as the diaphragm, massages your internal organs. The liver, stomach, and large intestine are the prime recipients of this gentle regular movement. Slow, deep breathing turns on the parasympathetic nervous system, which is responsible for all healing, proper digestion, hormonal balance, and a feeling of general well-being. Your mind can switch from a parasympathetic to a sympathetic state in the time it takes to form a stressful thought. And with regular practice, it can switch back again just as quickly.

Here's a simple, yet effective, breathing exercise you can do to get into the parasympathetic-dominant state.

Sit up straight or lie down on your back. Uncross your legs and arms, and close your eyes.

1. Take a deep breath and slowly blow it out through your mouth. Inhale deeply and slowly through your nose to a count of four. As you inhale, feel your abdomen and then your chest expand. Gently hold your breath for a count of four.

2. Then slowly exhale through your mouth to a count of eight. Repeat for at least five inhalations or up to twenty minutes at a time. Initially you may want to place your hands on your belly and chest to feel the expansion of each as you breathe. Set a timer. Falling asleep during this exercise indicates that you need more rest.

Start out slowly and be gentle with yourself. Like any skill, it takes practice to consistently reach a state of deep relaxation. To really feel the positive effects, you must practice getting into the parasympathetic state (also known as an alpha- or theta-brainwave state) daily. You don't need to meditate for hours at a time to feel better. You only need to do any form of skilled relaxation for twenty minutes, twice each day. If this sounds daunting, start with five minutes of deep breathing in the afternoon, or when transitioning between one activity and another, such as between work and returning home. Enter your relaxation time in your date book or schedule planner. Find a quiet place, set a timer, and work up to twenty minutes once a day; then add a second session. I encourage you to try many forms of relaxation techniques to find what works best for you. You can breathe deeply at your desk, when sitting in your parked car, or anywhere you can find a few moments of quiet.

If you are like many Americans, you have forgotten what it feels like to be totally relaxed. One way to rediscover the feeling of deep relaxation is to get six one-hour deep-tissue, full-body massages in the course of two weeks. It may sound expensive, but most certified massage therapists would be willing to give you a package deal. Once you have experienced how it feels to be really relaxed, you'll know when you've achieved a relaxed state through other means, such as deep breathing or meditation.

Another way to make sure you are achieving a state of relaxation is to use a biofeedback device. A wide variety is available, from the simple, nontechnical skin thermometer known as the Biodot to the more-technical breath-training videogame, *The Journey to Wild Divine*. These and other devices are good tools to get you started down the path of healing relaxation. Professional biofeedback therapists can also teach you how to relax deeply. (See the resources for more information.)

■ Case study: Jane

Jane, aged forty-one, came to my office with IBS symptoms. For the previous three years, she had experienced nausea, diarrhea, sharp abdominal pains, and bloating that increased by evening. Her symptoms had been worse in the last four months due to increased stress. She grew up on the standard American diet and had always had inhalant allergies. In the last ten years, she had improved her diet and done yoga occasionally, but the bloating, pain, and diarrhea episodes continued. She was taking a probiotic and a multivitamin, and needed to use her asthma inhaler every evening. Her energy was low, and her allergies were getting worse. A stool test showed low digestive enzymes; an unhealthful bacteria, *Clostridium difficile*; low levels of healthful bacteria; and very low IgA antibodies (an indication of long-term stress). She started the whole-food diet, avoiding all processed foods, and returned to daily yoga practice to help manage stress. With the addition of digestive enzymes and an HCl (hydrochloric acid) supplement, an antimicrobial herb, and adrenal support, she began feeling much better. Ten months later, her IBS symptoms were a thing of the past, as shown by her symptom survey results before and after the changes she made.

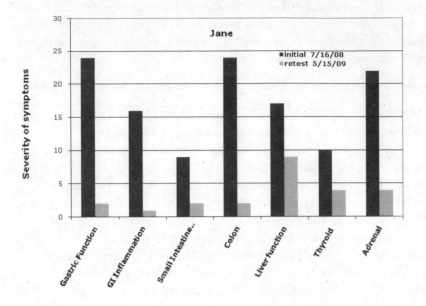

Figure 5.1   Jane's Symptom Survey Results

The Importance of Moderate Exercise

You don't need to train like an Olympic athlete to benefit from exercise. "Exercise" is just a name for deliberate and regular sustained movement. If diarrhea is one of your IBS symptoms and you are underweight or weak, or fatigue easily, movement is still important. Try to engage in nonstrenuous forms, such as gentle walking, qigong, tai chi, yoga, and stretching. If constipation is one of your IBS symptoms, moving will definitely help you improve frequency and ease of bowel movements. Start slowly; if you are sedentary and aren't used to any form of movement, start with five to ten minutes of walking or stretching. Gentle exercise like walking helps relieve IBS symptoms by improving circulation. Regular and continued movement of any kind (such as walking for thirty minutes) helps move wastes out of the tissues, balances the nervous system, and rhythmically massages your lower abdomen. Lifting your knees when you walk (marching) helps awaken and move a sluggish bowel.

Moving any part of your body alternately contracts and relaxes your muscles, which pushes the fluid between your cells, the *lymph fluid*, through channels in your body, known as *lymph vessels*, to be filtered and then returned to the blood-stream as plasma. Lymph carries wastes away from the cells, and is a pathway for white blood cells, which defend you against any pathogens. Unlike the blood, which the heart's action moves, the lymph moves only if you do. Removing waste from the tissues helps the digestive organs function properly.

Another good reason to engage in regular movement or exercise is to discharge stored stress. Part of the fight-or-flight response to stress is an automatic tensing of your muscles to get them ready to move, but if you neither fight nor flee, your muscles stay tense and ready. Exercise gives your muscles something to do and then allows them to relax more completely afterward. Exercise also increases the breathing rate and depth. If you can still converse while exercising, it's considered *aerobic* (with air) and your cells are getting more oxygen. If you are out of breath and can't converse during exercise, you are doing *anaerobic* (without enough air) exercise. When you engage in anaerobic exercise, your cells have too little oxygen, often resulting in fatigue afterward (Zhang et al. 2006). This fatigue is often the biggest reason you may not want to exercise consistently. Doing too much, too fast exceeds your aerobic capacity. Start slowly and don't push yourself to the point of breathlessness or exhaustion.

Enjoy exercise or some form of movement each day, but increase the duration or intensity very slowly. You need only thirty to forty minutes of exercise a day, and only three to five days a week, to benefit, and it need not be extreme. Pick a form of movement you enjoy. Walking is fine. Dancing by yourself to music in your home is easy and inexpensive, and qualifies as movement too. As you continue to exercise regularly and begin to feel better, you can increase the duration of your exercise by five minutes a week. Once you are exercising for thirty to forty minutes a day, you can increase your distance or intensity. Continue monitoring your breathing, and slow down if you can't talk (or softly sing) while exercising.

FOODS TO EMPHASIZE

What kind of food and how it's cooked make a big difference to someone with IBS. As Michael Pollan (2008, 1) so simply states in *In Defense of Food*, "Eat food, not too much, mostly plants." To adequately define food, this extremely articulate writer requires another 256 pages. I define food as seasonal, organic, unrefined, and local (SOUL foods), as nature provides them. Eating SOUL foods has helped my clients resolve many health issues. As with any process, the devil is in the details. But generally, fresh vegetables and natural, whole-food protein sources should constitute the basics of the IBS-friendly diet.

Our Ancestors' Diet

You can obtain every nutrient you need from what's called a *Paleolithic diet* (or *caveman diet*) consisting of fish or meat, and a variety of fresh seasonal vegetables (Cordain et al. 2005). If you have tested to make sure you aren't sensitive to them (see chapter 3), you can include fruit, grains, dairy, and beans in your diet, but they're not required for an IBS-therapeutic diet.

You can obtain all the nutrient-dense calories you need by eating plenty of vegetables, healthy fats, and high-quality proteins. The vegetables on this plan are nutrient dense and quite low in calories, compared to processed foods containing refined flour and sugar in the standard American diet, which provide many calories but few nutrients. Be sure to eat satisfying quantities of vegetables, as well as enough protein-rich foods, such as ocean fish, pasture-raised or organic eggs, poultry, and meats, with the natural fat therein, to maintain a healthy weight. (The recipes and menu plans will help with portion size.)

Many of my clients find they lose excess waistline inches as the gut heals. If you are underweight, make sure to eat several small to medium meals instead of three large meals a day, to avoid overtaxing your digestive capacity. Include foods high in healthy, natural fat, such as avocado, olives, and coconut, to help provide energy and fat-soluble vitamins. This book's recipes are meant as a rough guide; your "mileage" may vary. Experiment with what works best for you, and keep track of the foods that help you. You may discover you feel so good on this Paleolithic diet that you stay on it long term. Our ancestors were healthy and strong on a similar diet, and you can be too.

Preparing Foods to Fit Your Digestive Needs

In traditional Chinese medicine (TCM), constipation is considered a hot, dry condition, and diarrhea a cold, wet condition, so the opposite quality from foods balances each condition (Pitchford 2002). If you have diarrhea-predominant IBS, the TCM perspective emphasizes well-cooked vegetables and proteins because they are considered warming and easier to digest. Cooked foods are softer in texture and gentler to an irritated intestine. Cooking breaks down foods and makes many nutrients more bioavailable, but the heat of cooking can destroy some vitamins, so lower temperatures are better for retaining vitamins in cooked foods. Meats or beans slow cooked in a slow cooker or oven are more digestible and maintain more nutrients than faster, hotter cooking methods, such as broiling, frying, microwaving, or grilling. If constipation is your primary IBS symptom, cooling green salads, *cultured* (fermented) vegetables, or blended raw vegetable soups can gently stimulate a sluggish bowel. If you alternate between constipation and diarrhea, steamed vegetables and brothy soups are good choices, because cooked vegetables and liquids are more easily digested and all nutrients are more easily absorbed. Liquids and blended foods are gentler to your sensitive digestive system.

The Power of Green Foods

Green foods are exceptionally healing for the gut, the liver, and the rest of the body. Green is the color of most plant life, yet some people avoid green foods (with the exception of a little lettuce, lime-gelatin desserts, or green beer!). Our ancestors included a variety of plants in their diet. Green vegetables, especially dark, leafy greens, provide a powerhouse of the nutrients you need for healing. Examples of the healing green foods most helpful to IBS sufferers are kale, collard greens, mustard greens, bok choy, turnip greens, spinach, chard, beet greens, amaranth greens, mint, basil, cilantro, parsley, purslane, arugula, romaine lettuce, and green-leaf lettuce..Greens are a low-calorie source of necessary nutrients. Some of their known nutrients are; chlorophyll; most vitamins, including beta-carotene and vitamins C, E, K, and B complex; antioxidants, including alpha-lipoic acid; a balance of minerals (especially magnesium, potassium, calcium, and iron); some essential fatty acids (which help reduce inflammation); a little protein; lots of fiber; and lesser known but very important plant nutrients. Science is just beginning to understand the role these plant nutrients, also known as *phytonutrients*, provide. Some health-building phytonutrients found in green plant foods are bioflavonoids, anthocyanins, indoles, isothiocyanates, and sulforaphanes.

Green plants contain chlorophyll, the pigment responsible for photosynthesis. Without this energy-producing pigment, life on earth would be very different. The darker the green color, the more chlorophyll the plant contains. Chlorophyll is very similar to hemoglobin, the red protein in our blood, differing by only one atom. Hemoglobin contains one atom of iron as its central mineral, whereas chlorophyll has magnesium. Magnesium is a mineral that's an essential cofactor of many of our metabolic processes, including those required for optimal digestion, energy production, muscle relaxation, healing, and pain relief, and green plant foods provide it to us. Chlorophyll cleanses the breath and the entire digestive tract, and helps the liver detoxify. Adding several servings of green leafy vegetables (cooked or raw) to your daily diet is one of the fastest and most reliable ways to improve gut health.

The Power of Foods from the Sea

Not many Americans eat seaweed, and some dislike fish, but foods from the sea are rich in many of our necessary trace minerals, which have washed into our oceans over the millennia. Seaweed has been valued by cultures from the Japanese along the Pacific shores to the Europeans along the North Atlantic Ocean. Inland peoples traded for the valuable sea salt, fish, and seaweed they knew kept them healthy. You may currently eat extracts of seaweed in the form of MSG, agar, and carrageenan in processed foods, but you'll want to avoid these since they are chemically concentrated extracts rather than whole foods. Instead, get all the sea has to offer by sprinkling granules of the purple seaweed dulse on your foods instead of salt, wrapping snacks sushi-style in nori sheets, and eating EFA-rich cold-water ocean fish, such as sardines, salmon, cod, and halibut. There's a list of low-contaminant fish that aren't overfished online at www.edf.org (type "seafood selector" into the search field). Hand-harvested seaweed from clean coastlines is recommended (see the resources).

A No-Fun Fungus

If you have IBS, there's a strong possibility that you have an intestinal imbalance, or overgrowth, of the yeast and fungus *Candida albicans* (see chapter 2), a condition known as candidiasis. If you have ever taken a course of powerful broad-spectrum antibiotics or had to take any antibiotic for more than two weeks, you probably have this imbalance. These antibiotics kill most types of bacteria, but not yeasts, so the good bacteria that keep yeasts from proliferating are destroyed, allowing yeast to grow out of control. Yeasts love sugar, fruit, and starch, so a diet containing these will feed the yeasts, resulting in many IBS symptoms in the process. An excess of candida creates alcohol, acetic acid, formaldehyde, acetaldehyde, and a multitude of irritating compounds as its waste products. The very fine roots (*hyphae* and *pseudohyphae*) (Fujita, Tokunaga, and Inoue 1971) of a yeast or fungus burrow into the intestinal lining, seeking food and creating intestinal hyperpermeability, or leaky gut (Spiller et al. 2000). Our body tries to defend against this invader by creating antibodies to attack its proteins. The antibodies you produce against the kind of fungus in your intestine may also recognize other kinds of fungus, such as mushrooms (which are actually large, edible fungi), nutritional yeast, baker's yeast, or foods fermented using yeast or fungi, meaning these foods can also become irritating. To find out if you have candidiasis or another fungal overgrowth, get a stool test from an alternative lab that can identify gut-flora imbalances. Standard labs don't reliably or accurately identify candidiasis. (See the resources for recommended labs.)

SOME FUN FUNGI: MEDICINAL MUSHROOMS

Chinese medicinal mushrooms (shiitake, maitake, reishi, and others) have been eaten or used in tea for centuries to improve health. Mushrooms are low-calorie sources of B vitamins, trace minerals, amino acids, and fiber. Shiitake, maitake, and reishi mushrooms support the immune system, helping to defend you from harmful invaders. However, everyone's reaction to fungi is different. The only way to tell if you can use medicinal mushrooms is to try them and see how you react. If medicinal mushrooms don't bother your digestive system, you may find they are a tasty way to help strengthen your immune system, and help your digestive system heal and function normally again. Include some medicinal mushrooms in soups, stews, and sautéed vegetables.

Vegetable Fiber Is Gentle to the Irritable Bowel

Much controversy exists around using fiber when you have IBS. Generally, if diarrhea is your primary IBS symptom, you need to avoid wheat bran and other supplemental fiber because they are often too rough or may be allergenic for the sensitive bowel. You need a natural ratio of soluble to insoluble fiber, which a variety of vegetables contains, especially dark-green leafy vegetables, crunchy and cruciferous vegetables, such as cabbage, broccoli, Brussels sprouts, and cauliflower, and stalks, such as celery, asparagus, leeks, scallions, and fennel. Cooking vegetables in a soup or stew softens their fibers and liberates the minerals and vitamins into the broth, increasing the availability and absorbability of all the nutrients. Soups and broths are traditional comfort foods as well. If constipation is your primary IBS symptom, it's likely you're not consuming enough fiber-rich foods and fluids, or you may be sensitive to a particular type of food you are eating, such as wheat.

Flaxseeds and chia and psyllium seeds are all sources of soluble fiber (mucilage) which may benefit some people with IBS and harm others. (See chapter 4 for more info on fiber and what kind to eat to enhance your digestive process and avoid harmful bacteria.)

Flaxseeds (also known as *linseeds*) are the seeds of the *Linum usitatissimum* plant, a native of India and the Mediterranean. Approximately 57 percent of the oil in flaxseeds is alpha-linolenic acid, an essential omega-3 fatty acid that's important for reducing inflammation and improving healing. You can add between one teaspoon and one tablespoon a day of the filtered oil as a dressing on greens or in smoothies. Remember to store flaxseed oil in the freezer (it thickens but still pours) to prevent this delicate omega-3 oil from oxidizing or becoming rancid too quickly. If flaxseed oil tastes bitter, it's rancid, and you shouldn't consume it. Filtered flaxseed oil contains zero fiber. If you're not sensitive to the fiber in the seeds, you can use unfiltered flaxseed oil or add one or two tablespoons of ground flaxseed to a smoothie to thicken it and to provide essential omega-3 fatty acids.

Native to Mexico, chia seeds, *Salvia hispanica*, were a staple food in the Aztec culture for centuries. (Yes, these are the same chia seeds that are sprouted on the terra-cotta Chia Pets, though those may contain chemicals and aren't for human consumption.) Chia is another seed that's very rich in alpha-linolenic acid. When added to liquids, the soluble fiber surrounding each chia seed absorbs water and swells, forming a slippery, gelatinous mass, reminiscent of tapioca but with a slightly crunchy, nutty taste. You can eat sprouted chia instead of alfalfa sprouts. You can use ground chia seeds as a nutritious whole-food thickener and add it to baked goods to improve the fiber content. A mix of chia seeds and coconut water is a healthier version of *chia fresca*, a popular drink in Central America.

Psyllium-seed husk, the outer seed coat of the plant *Plantago ovata*, is rich in mucilage and is an often-suggested treatment for constipation. Plain psyllium-seed husk is available at health food stores and is the major ingredient of many bowel-cleansing formulas. The plain husks are preferable to the commercially processed versions that contain potentially irritating artificial colors, flavors, and sweeteners. Psyllium-seed husk is very inexpensive, and can be added to smoothies and other recipes to thicken them without adding any flavor of its own. For those who aren't bothered by soluble fiber or mucilage, it relieves constipation, because the fiber holds onto water in the stool, and it can also help firm the stool if you have mild diarrhea.

Be very careful when using grains or seeds as sources of fiber. Many people with IBS are actually allergic to or intolerant of many grains and seeds, and products that include them. Whole grains are very high in insoluble fiber (roughage), and the nutrients they contain are more difficult to absorb unless the grains are properly soaked, sprouted, or fermented. Consuming fiber with inadequate water can cause constipation. Always add at least three times as much liquid to any dry fiber-rich food to prevent formation of blockages in the large intestine. This book's recipes are designed with the right amounts of liquid and kinds of fiber needed to benefit the irritable bowel.

Include Cultured Foods

Cultured foods are natural sources of beneficial bacteria. Every world culture has its culture—that is, some food that it ferments (or *cultures*) to help maintain good health. Before refrigeration, fermentation was a very important way to store food safely. Allowing foods to naturally ferment, or sour, is a natural way to preserve food for extended periods. Adding salt, lemon juice, whey, or vinegar (whey and vinegar are created by fermentation) creates an environment that encourages many healthful bacteria (such as *lactobacillus*) to make lactic acid, which prevents harmful microorganisms from growing. Eating fermented or cultured foods promotes the growth of healthful bacteria in our intestines. Fermented foods have been popular for centuries in various parts of the globe. Yogurt and kefir are eaten in the Mediterranean. Sauerkraut, cheese, and pickled cucumbers (commonly known as pickles), peppers, beets, and turnips are popular in Eastern Europe. Asian cuisine includes kimchi, pickled ginger, tempeh, tamari, and miso. Latin America has a version of sauerkraut called *cortido*, and salsa was originally cultured. Fermented taro root is known as *poi* in the Polynesian islands. Even ketchup, mustard, and chutney were originally fermented. Letting healthful bacteria break down foods for us makes digestion easier, increases the nutritional value of the food, allows the food to keep longer, and often improves flavor (Katz 2003).

Unfortunately most commercial sauerkraut and yogurt are pasteurized, so they don't contain the healthful bacteria that can help heal the gut. Choose brands listed in the resources, and look for "raw" or "contains live cultures" on the labels (Rani and Khetarpaul 1998). Better yet, make your own to ensure they are full of healthful bacteria and don't contain any ingredients to which you are sensitive. Chapter 8 shows you how to culture sauerkraut, seeds, and even grains to make them more nourishing and digestible. For many more cultured recipes, read *Wild Fermentation: The Flavor, Nutrition, and Craft of Live-Culture Foods*, by Sandor E. Katz (Chelsea Green, 2003). Please be advised that raw foods can contain all kinds of bacteria, so immune-compromised patients should proceed with caution (Katz 2003; Schmid 2009).

FOODS TO AVOID

Eliminating irritating foods and food-like substances isn't easy in our society, but you have to do it to heal from IBS. It's important to remember that the gut is not a garbage disposal and shouldn't be treated as one. Treat your body as you would an expensive sports car. You wouldn't put poor-quality, contaminated gasoline or used oil in the finest automobile and expect it to run optimally.

Yet many people expect the digestive system to function asymptomatically and efficiently, even though they eat refined, processed, and generally poor-quality food. You get what you pay for, and poor digestive health can be the ultimate price of eating processed food. Whole food is simple and powerful, but it must be fresh to provide optimum health, so it has a short shelf life and can cost a bit more.

As discussed in chapter 3, it's important to identify your trigger foods, using the elimination diet with provocative food testing or a food-allergy blood test. However, there are some substances everyone needs to avoid to regain or maintain good health: generally, refined carbohydrates, and specifically, sugars; industrialized fats such as hydrogenated oils; generally, chemicals; and poor-quality proteins, such as isolated soy protein and hydrolyzed vegetable protein. Protein powders can be damaged or contaminated during chemical isolation processing. You also need to avoid irritating substances such as caffeine, chocolate, tobacco, and alcohol, as well as any foods with chemical additives.

Carefully read the ingredients lists (the very fine print) on all packaged foods. Avoid any food with a large list of ingredients, especially if it contains complex chemical names. Again, you shouldn't need a chemistry degree to figure out what's in your food. Some ingredients to avoid include: artificial sweeteners, such as aspartame (NutraSweet, Equal), sucralose (Splenda), and saccharine (Sweet'N Low); flavor stimulants such as monosodium glutamate (MSG), which may be labeled as "natural flavor"; preservatives such as butylated hydroxyanisole (BHA) and butylated hydroxytoluene (BHT); and artificial flavorings (vanillin and many others) and colorings (including FD&C yellow 5 or red 40, and benzidine). The sweeteners xylitol, sorbitol, and mannitol are known to induce diarrhea in sensitive individuals, especially when consumed in large amounts, such as in candy or baked goods. These and many other chemically derived ingredients have been linked to IBS (Antico et al. 1989). Some scientists feel the FDA has not adequately evaluated many of these chemical additives for human consumption (Mercola and Pearsall 2006), and they have not been tested in combination with one another.

Refined Carbohydrates

White sugar, white flour, white rice, white pasta, cornstarch, peeled potatoes, fruit juice, high-fructose corn syrup, and pearled barley are common examples of refined carbohydrates (Davis 1970; Loiselle 1993; Price 1945). To get what many people think of as "normal" cereal, pasta, rice, and breads, food-processing companies start with the whole grain, then remove the bran and germ, which contain the majority of the vitamins and minerals, and then grind, sift, and bleach the remaining inner portion, or *endosperm*, which is mostly starch. They do this to give the "food" a longer shelf life. After all this processing, no self-respecting microbe will touch it. Eating processed food does nothing to extend your life. Even peeled potatoes have lost their most nutritious part, the skin.

Refining and processing of food removes the fiber along with most of the vitamins and minerals. White flour has lost 72 percent of the vitamin B6, 86 percent of the vitamin E, 66 percent of the folic acid, 80 percent of the thiamin and niacin, 60 percent of the calcium, and 85 percent of the magnesium normally in whole wheat (Schroeder 1971). Because these refined products don't contain the fiber and nutrients the body requires to metabolize carbohydrates, the body uses nutrients from its own reserves. According to Ronald Schmid, ND, in *Traditional Foods Are Your Best Medicine* (1997) (and many other holistic nutritionists), continual consumption of refined carbohydrates can lead to nutrient depletion and disease. Sugar and other highly refined carbohydrates can be considered anti-nutrients.

SUGAR

Sugar is both psychologically and physically addictive (Avena, Rada, and Hoebel 2008). According to medical definitions, a substance is addictive if it induces a pleasant state or relieves distress; causes long-term chemical changes in the brain; leads to adaptive changes in the brain that trigger tolerance, physical dependence, and uncontrollable cravings; and causes dependence, so that abstaining is difficult and creates severe physical and mental reactions. Sugar has been shown to cause all of these reactions (Colantuoni et al. 2002). Parasites and pathogens thrive on sugar (Gittleman 2001). If you have IBS, it's important to avoid all forms of isolated sugar, including brown sugar, raw sugar, turbinado sugar, Sucanat, sucrose, fructose, dextrose, glucose (or any substance that ends in "-ose"), maltodextrin, high-fructose corn syrup, corn syrup, agave nectar, barley malt, rice syrup, molasses, cane sugar, evaporated cane juice, beet sugar, and even more-natural forms of sweeteners, such as date sugar, honey, and maple syrup. If this sounds impossible, don't despair. Start by reading all food labels. If you can't give up sugar "cold turkey," take it one day at a time, slowly reducing your intake. You will also need to eliminate the processed foods that contain hidden sugar, which are many and increasing each day as our food becomes "new and improved." Manufacturers often add sugar in a multitude of forms to make the food irresistible, so read all ingredient labels carefully. If some form of sugar is among the first three ingredients, that food is a dessert.

Here are five simple guidelines for avoiding sugar and refined carbohydrates:

- Eat all your foods as they are found in nature, for example, fresh, natural, unprocessed vegetables, fruit, grains, beans, nuts, and seeds.

- Read ingredient labels. Avoid ingredients that end in "-ose" or "-ol" or have sugars (or chemicals) in them. If some form of sugar is among the first three ingredients, don't eat it.

- Don't drink soda or fruit drinks. Soda has quite a lot of sugar (about 12 teaspoons per 12 ounces) or contains artificial sweeteners. Fruit juice has had nutrient-rich fiber removed, so it isn't whole and can raise blood sugar too rapidly. Instead, try sparkling mineral water with a squeeze of lemon or lime, or herbal tea.

- Don't eat foods labeled "fat free." Often even more sugar or other refined carbohydrates are added to make up for the reduced fat.

- Don't add sugar or artificial sweeteners to what you drink or eat. Get rid of your sugar bowl and those silly packets. Eliminate sucralose (Splenda), aspartame (Equal), and saccharin (Sweet'N Low) from your diet. Since sugar substitutes may actually promote weight gain (Hampton 2008), eating whole food, which satisfies nutritional needs, is a much better way to lose weight.

SPECIFIC SUGARS AND STARCHES: DISACCHARIDES AND AMYLOSE

According to Elaine Gottschall in her book *Breaking the Vicious Cycle* (1994), some sugars and starches irritate the intestines because some people have difficulty digesting these particular types of carbohydrates. When eaten by people with damage to the beginning of the small intestine, the intact carbohydrates travel farther along the digestive tract, becoming food for harmful bacteria that leave waste products that contribute to problems such as IBS and even IBD. The starch to restrict is *amylose*, which is in grains, starchy root vegetables, bread, and pasta. The sugars to restrict are *disaccharides*, namely, sucrose (table sugar), maltose (all grains), and lactose (in most dairy). Not everyone is sensitive to all of these foods, but many individuals with gastrointestinal problems improve dramatically when they remove these sugars and starches from their diet.

According to Gottschall (Ibid.), the foods with excessive *disaccharides* or *amylose* are:

Agar	Cellulose gum	Mannitol
Agave	Cereals (all)	Mucilaginous vegetables and herbs (all)
Alcohol (most)	Chewing gum	Plantains
Algae	Chickory root	Potatoes
Aloe vera	Chocolate	Protein powder
Arrowroot	Coffee	Psyllium husks
Astragalus	Corn	Rice
Bean sprouts	Cornstarch	Seaweed
Beans (most)	Dairy (unless fermented more than sixty days)	Sorbitol
Bee pollen	Fructo-oligo saccharides (FOS)	Soy (all forms)
Bitter gourd	Fruit juice (all)	Starchy roots (all)
Bouillon cubes	Grain beverages	Starchy vegetables (most)
Bread	Grains and flour (all)	Sugar (all)
Burdock root	Guar gum	Water chestnuts
Buttermilk	Jicama	Xylitol
Canned vegetables (all)	Licorice	Yeast
Carob	Lunch meats (all)	Yogurt (unless home-made and fermented twenty-four hours or more)
Carrageenan		

Industrialized Fats

The kinds of fats you consume can directly affect your IBS symptoms (Kilkins et al. 2004). Industrialized, processed fats generally aren't beneficial for digestive health, and are even worse for those with IBS. Just as food-processing companies want to increase shelf life of breads and cereals, they also want to process fats so they don't become rancid, which contributes to stale flavors in baked goods. If a food doesn't taste fresh, it won't sell, which is why the food industry refines and hydrogenates oils. Even though trans fats have been reduced in processed foods, hydrogenated fats are found in nearly every processed food at the grocery, including peanut butter, salad dressings, chicken nuggets, French fries, doughnuts, coffee whitener, and, of course, margarine. As mentioned previously, if a serving contains less than half a gram of trans-fatty acids, manufacturers are allowed to claim that it contains "zero trans fats per serving." Hydrogenated fats are artificially saturated fats. (Trans fats are unsaturated but still harmful.) Hydrogenation of oils damages sensitive essential fatty acids, creating harmful free radicals, and removes the fat-soluble vitamins A, D, E, and K (Enig 2000). The industrialized processing of fats creates many and varied health problems (Ravnskov 2000). Since the introduction of hydrogenated fats in the early 1900s, we have increasingly included them in our diet, and overall health has suffered greatly since then. Hydrogenation produces the saturated fats that many studies have shown to harm the cardiovascular, nervous, immune, and digestive systems (Enig 2000). The percentage of naturally saturated fats consumed has decreased in the last hundred years, while consumption of the unnatural hydrogenated and refined fats has increased, along with chronic health problems (Ibid.).

Poor-Quality Proteins

The usability and digestibility of proteins declines when they are damaged or contaminated. Damage can occur from excess or prolonged heat, time, oxygen, hydrolysis by acids, catalysis by enzymes, radiation (including microwave), or strong alkalis (such as lye) (Millán, Brito, and Hevia 1984; Nakamura et al. 1994; de Pomerai et al. 2003). Contamination was in the global news in 2007, when it was discovered that feed and feed ingredients from China contained the plastic melamine to falsely increase the measure of protein in the feed. Baby formula was also found to contain the contaminant melamine after nearly three hundred thousand babies became ill and at least six died (Martin 2007).

Protein isolates (soy, rice, whey, and others) are found in protein bars, baby food formula, vegetarian meat substitutes, supplements, and many foods, and they're created using solvents, such as hexane, acids, and other chemicals. Though manufacturers try to remove all of these chemicals, traces remain and can affect how you digest, absorb, and metabolize. These chemicals negatively affect the liver (Rabovsky, Judy, and Pailes 1986). Consume proteins as whole foods you can recognize, such as beans, nuts, fish, eggs, and meat.

Foods with Chemicals

We are surrounded by 5 to 7 million different kinds of man-made chemicals, and 400 million tons are produced worldwide per year (International Labour Organization 2006). From food, cars, furniture, clothing, household items, paints, pesticides, detergents, and cleaners to hair- and body-care products, you are exposed to a chemical soup that you were never meant to encounter and that your body has to work to eliminate. According to the training booklet *Chemicals in the Workplace*, by the International Labour Organization (Ibid.), and *Pollution in People*, a report by the Toxic-Free Legacy Coalition (Schreder 2006), hazardous additives in food, cosmetics, and consumer goods enter the body via ingestion, inhalation, and skin absorption. You can't detoxify and eliminate all of these industrial chemicals, so they accumulate in all of your tissues from the time you are born—in your lungs, fatty tissue, blood, liver, kidneys, brain, bone marrow, and skin. The accumulation of heavy metals, such as mercury and lead, is widespread in humans (Mozaffarian and Rimm 2006). Mercury and other contaminants contained in fish and seafood may be why so may people are sensitive to these otherwise-healthy foods.

According to the World Health Organization's International Programme on Chemical Safety, foods contain a multitude of toxic chemicals, many of which we can and should avoid to improve health (WHO Task Group on Environmental Health Criteria for Principles for Modelling Dose-Response for the Risk Assessment of Chemicals 2009). At the very least, you can limit your exposure to these toxins by making sure they aren't in your foods or body-care products. Avoid all foods containing added chemicals. Read all ingredient labels carefully, including the fine print. Every day you avoid a chemical exposure, you decrease your chances of harming your digestive system and the rest of your body. Toxic chemicals, even in small amounts, can and do irritate the bowel.

Avoid packaged foods to begin with. Food requires preservatives only if it's not fresh. Ripe vegetables and fruit don't need to be dyed or have artificial colors added. Food dyes are made from petrochemicals that, though toxic in large amounts, are assumed to be harmless in small quantities. For a list of food additives, the Center for Science in the Public Interest (CSPI) has a frequently updated website (cspinet.org). For information on chemicals in cosmetics, read *Dying to Look Good: The Disturbing Truth About What's Really in Your Cosmetics, Toiletries, and Personal Care Products*, by Christine Hoza Farlow (Kiss for Health Publishing, 2005). See the resources for more information.

In addition to added chemicals, many plants create toxins as protection against insects and other pests. Some people are quite sensitive to these compounds, either because their total load of toxins is already quite high or because of a genetic predisposition toward sensitivity to these particular chemicals. Some of these chemicals are:

- Solanine, as found in plants in the nightshade family (Solanaceae), such as tomato, potato, eggplant, pepper, tomatillo, pimento, cayenne, paprika, and tobacco

- Lectins in most grains, especially wheat germ, and beans, especially kidney beans, soybeans, and lima beans (D'Mello 2003)

- Oxalic acid in rhubarb, sorrel, star fruit (carambola), black pepper, parsley, poppy seed, amaranth, spinach, chard, beets, cocoa, and chocolate

BENEFICIAL HERBS

You can use many herbs and spices to help heal IBS, either singly—as *simples*—or in combinations. A study reported in the British medical journal *Lancet* showed that professionally prescribed Chinese herbs, such as *Xiao Yao Wan* and *Tong Xie Yao Fang*, significantly improved IBS (Senior 1998). Herbs can have a powerful action on the human body if they are used in the correct form, the right dosage and frequency, and the appropriate combination. See an acupuncturist for the proper herbal remedy for you.

Listed next are the most commonly used herbs and their actions. As with foods, you may need a four-day rotation of herbs to avoid developing a sensitivity to them.

Soothing Herbs

You can use these herbs in recipes or make them into a therapeutic tea.

- Anise: mild sedative; reduces gas and cramps; regulates digestion

- Caraway: for colic and indigestion; stimulates gastric juices (May et al. 1996)

- Chamomile: antispasmodic, antimicrobial; makes a relaxing tea (Hobbs 1992)

- Fennel: reduces bloating and gas (Ibid.)

- Ginger: relieves nausea, motion sickness, and cramps

- Oregano: antispasmodic; relieves nausea

- Peppermint: antispasmodic, analgesic, antifungal (May et al. 1996)

- Schizandra: Chinese berry that regulates the GI tract; use in tea

- Trifala (or triphala): a combination of three Ayurvedic fruits— *Terminalia chebula* (haritaki), *Terminalia bellerica* (bahera), and *Emblica officinalis* (amla)—to regulate the bowel. Start with a quarter teaspoon of powdered trifala twice daily, and gradually increase the amount until you find the optimal dosage to move the bowels without causing diarrhea.

Antimicrobial Herbs

Ancient peoples have always consumed herbs to eliminate harmful parasites and pests. You should do the same once or twice a year to cleanse your colon of potential and actual parasites. Spring and fall are the traditional times to use these herbs. If you suspect you have an invader, or if a stool test shows this, it's important to eliminate it without damaging your digestive tract with harsh chemicals, such as antibiotics or fungicides. Some bacteria have become resistant to the antibiotics currently available, because antibiotics kill the weak ones, leaving the strong to multiply. Thankfully bacteria are usually still susceptible to a rotation of herbal capsules and strong teas.

Berberine: Herbs containing berberine, such as Oregon grape root, barberry, goldenseal root, golden thread (or coptis), and yellow dock, are all antiparasitic (Subbaiah and Amin 1967), antifungal, and antibacterial (Vanderhoof et al. 1999). You can take these herbs as a tea or tincture or in capsules or tablets, three times a day. Berberine has been shown to relieve diarrhea and has been used against bacteria, yeasts, viruses, and amoebas (Kaneda, Tanaka, and Saw 1990; Rabbani et al. 1987; Gupte 1975). Contained in several bitter, yellow roots, it helps the liver detoxify and helps regulate blood sugar and cholesterol. Goldenseal is now endangered, so use Oregon grape root instead. Avoid all berberine-containing herbs during pregnancy.

Oil of Oregano: Oil of oregano contains the substance *carvacrol*, which inhibits the fungus candida, a possible cause of IBS (Murray and Pizzorno 1998). Adding oregano to foods is a pleasant way to help combat intestinal infections, although you can obtain therapeutic amounts only from capsules. Other volatile oils, such as peppermint, rosemary, and thyme, are also useful antimicrobials. These oils are available to the small and large intestines when administered as enteric-coated capsules. An effective dose is 0.2 to 0.4 milliliter twice daily between meals (Ibid.).

Pau d'Arco: The inner bark of a South American tree, pau d'arco (*Tabebuia impetiginosa*) is an antifungal and immune-enhancing herb that tonifies the gastrointestinal tract. Two to three cups a day of a cold infusion of one ounce of the herb per quart of water for one month is generally helpful in fighting yeast and other fungal overgrowths that can affect the gut (Haas 1992). Capsules are also available.

Stevia: The antifungal South American herb stevia is a great substitute for artificial sweeteners while you're on the IBS diet (or anytime). Though a hundred times sweeter than sugar, it doesn't raise the blood sugar. Available as a powder or tincture, it can be used to taste, but the dried, powdered leaf tastes better, has less aftertaste, and still contains minerals and fiber. Avoid stevia extracts that contain FOS or dextrose. FOS is a type of soluble fiber that can irritate the intestines, because it can feed klebsiella bacteria.

Grapefruit Seed Extract (GSE): The bitter GSE liquid is said to kill all kinds of microbes and fungi, including the "good guys." Dilute it before using internally or topically. Mix five to fifteen drops in five ounces of water or herbal tea, two to five times daily, either with or between meals. It's also available in tablet form. There are no apparent side effects, even with long-term use (Galland 1995), but if you use GSE internally, be sure to replace your healthful bacteria by eating cultured foods, taking probiotic supplements (described in the next section), or both.

Olive Leaf Extract: Olive leaf extract has been used throughout recorded history as a remedy for bacterial, viral, fungal, and protozoan infections (Juven, Henis, and Jacoby 1972). The bitter phytophenols in olive leaf contain *oleuropein*, which has been shown to interfere with the reproduction of microbes and to increase the effectiveness of our protective white blood cells (Ibid.).

ADDITIONAL SUPPLEMENTS TO AID IBS

Here are a few natural substances to use when symptoms strike as you change your diet. These supplements can make it easier for you to function, as well as provide long-lasting support for gut functioning.

Detoxifiers

Bentonite Clay (*Montmorillonite*): A traditional treatment for toxicity used all over the world for centuries, clay swells like a sponge when wet and holds onto toxins electrostatically to harmlessly eliminate them in the stool. Because it has the ability to bind stools, clay is a remedy for diarrhea. (One popular over-the-counter remedy was originally a mixture of clay and the soluble fiber pectin, but now contains bismuth subsalicylate.) You can purchase bentonite, or montmorillonite, clay in wet or dry form. The wet form, sold as Sonne's #7, is easy to use but more expensive and less portable. Dry clay is available at health food stores or online and used this way: In about half a cup of warm (not hot) water, sprinkle one teaspoon of the clay powder. Don't stir yet, or dry lumps will occur. Allow the clay to get wet and settle to the bottom of the cup, which takes about ten minutes. When the clay is completely wet and has fallen to the bottom of the cup, stir the clay water, crushing any lumps. Drink the whole clay-water mixture. It has a neutral taste and pleasant, smooth texture. It should begin to help reduce pain, swelling, and gas within twenty to thirty minutes. Remember to stay hydrated by drinking plenty of water for easier bowel movements.

Charcoal Capsules: Powdered, activated charcoal acts much like clay by absorbing all kinds of chemical toxins (and foul odors) in the digestive tract and allowing them to pass out of the body harmlessly in the stool. In fact, charcoal is used as an emergency treatment for some kinds of poisonings. Follow the instructions on the charcoal product you use, but generally one teaspoon mixed in four to eight ounces of water, or two or three capsules, is a sufficient dosage to bring relief. Charcoal may darken the stool temporarily.

Gut Rebuilders

L-Glycine: L-glycine, the smallest amino acid, is a precursor to the powerful antioxidant glutathione and is required in the liver for detoxification. Without it, toxins can build up in the body and cause irritation in many tissues, especially the intestines. The body can make it, and it's found in many foods containing protein. Because it's a major component of cartilage, bone broth is an exemplary source. You can use one to three grams a day as a supplement in capsules or powder.

L-Glutamine: L-glutamine, another amino acid, is also a precursor to glutathione and is a fuel source for the cells lining the intestines. It has long been used intravenously in Europe to improve the integrity of the intestinal lining of those who have had a major injury, surgery, an infection, or radiation. It stimulates collagen formation necessary for wound healing. Take one teaspoon dissolved in water or tea, one to three times a day on an empty stomach. Some people report that L-glutamine makes them feel wired or causes a racing mind. Feeling overstimulated by L-glutamine indicates a deficiency of B vitamins, particularly B3 and B6, so you may want to eat more foods containing them.

Probiotics

Probiotics are supplementary preparations containing healthful bacteria. *Lactobacillus acidophilus, Bifidobacterium lactis, Bifidobacterium infantis, Lactobacillus plantarum, Lactobacillus casei*, and *Saccharomyces boulardii* are just a few of the more than four hundred species of beneficial organisms your large intestine needs for proper functioning. When bacterial imbalances occur, you can experience the IBS symptoms of gas, bloating, pain, and diarrhea or constipation. The natural world is teeming with both healthful and harmful bacteria. In a healthy digestive system, the good bacteria outnumber the bad, preventing the bad bacteria from proliferating. Since food moves through the digestive system every day that you eat something, bacteria get pushed out of the intestine with every bowel movement and must be replaced daily. You can replace helpful bacteria by eating cultured foods, such as sauerkraut, yogurt, and kefir, which contain live organisms. With IBS, you often need supplemental forms of these healthful organisms (Faber, Rigden, and Lukaczer 2005), but take care to ensure that the supplement contains them in large-enough numbers, or you'll waste much money and time (Hogg 2006). Look for supplements containing the recommended 10 billion live organisms per dosage (Camilleri 2008), and keep probiotic supplements refrigerated to ensure efficacy. (See the resources for recommended suppliers of supplements.)

Digestive Enzymes

Many circumstances bring about the need for digestive enzymes. When you are under stress, as you age, or even when you overeat and exceed your digestive capacity, taking additional digestive enzymes as supplements can help break down foods, making them more absorbable and less irritating. When food is absorbed more completely, the harmful bacteria in the large intestine have less to eat, so fewer gases and toxins are produced, reducing bowel irritation. If you have gas after you eat, even after slowing down and chewing thoroughly, you may want to try digestive bitters (a solution of bitter and aromatic herbs) to increase your production of digestive secretions. If that doesn't help, you may want to experiment with enzymes. If you have indigestion after eating meat or other protein, you may also need to supplement with hydrochloric acid tablets in the form of betaine hydrochloride. As with most things, you get what you pay for. Enzymes are damaged easily by heat and time. The most effective brands contain a mix of protease, lipase, amylase, and pancreas extract. (See the resources for preferred suppliers of supplements.)

There are many ways to improve your digestion and reduce IBS symptoms. You can start by removing all irritants, whether foods you are sensitive to, non-foods with chemical additives, or harmful bacteria, yeasts, or parasites. You can add bitters or digestive enzymes and HCl to improve digestion and thus reduce the painful and embarrassing gas that builds up when food ferments in the gut. You can make sure you are eating a wide variety of seasonal, organic, unrefined, and local (SOUL) foods to provide you with adequate nutrients all the time. You can reintroduce healthful bacteria to your digestive system by using naturally cultured foods and, if necessary, probiotic supplements. And you can repair any damage done by years of imbalance with skilled relaxation and specific healing nutrients.

6

Kitchen Setup for Simplified Cooking

To do any job, you need the proper tools. To make it easier and faster to make delicious meals and snacks without spending all of your time and energy, having some basic kitchen equipment on hand is an absolute necessity. Get the best-quality tools you can afford. You don't need to get the most expensive brand. Regular department stores and even hardware stores often have sales on high-quality items. Or try some of my favorite sources—secondhand stores, yard sales, and estate sales—for durable kitchen tools.

Necessary Tools

- A place to work, such as a counter or table, free of paper, books, and debris.

- A working stove and oven, preferably gas, but electric will do.

- Wooden cutting board. The plastic ones are shown to be less hygienic (Park and Cliver 1997), and who wants plastic bits in their food?

- Large chopping knife, preferably high quality. The better stainless-steel knives stay sharp longer and are more comfortable to use. Dull knives slip and cause accidents.

- Small paring knife.

- Serrated knife; especially good for cutting tomatoes without cutting yourself.

- Cast-iron skillets, nine- and six-inch with lids. Avoid nonstick coatings, because they flake off into the food, disrupting hormones, and are toxic when overheated (Fairley et al. 2007). Iron distributes heat evenly, and food won't stick if the pan is properly seasoned: heat the pan first, and then add the oil.

- Glass casserole dishes for cooking, serving, and storing foods. Glass insulates and is excellent for slow, even cooking. Avoid heating plastic containers (as in a microwave) to reduce your exposure to toxins.

- Stainless-steel stockpot with lid and steamer baskets.

- Steamer, if your stockpot doesn't have steamer baskets.

- Stainless-steel pans with lids. Three-ply (or five-ply) stainless steel over an aluminum core distributes heat well to prevent burning, and is lightweight.

- Measuring cups and measuring spoons. These help you reliably reproduce recipes.

- Blender (heavy-duty preferred) for sauces, dressings, smoothies, and soups.

- Unbleached parchment paper for drying nuts and seeds and making crackers.

Optional Tools

- Food processor; very handy for large chopping jobs or blended soups.

- Slow cooker or Crock-Pot; great for stews and soups, quick and easy to set up. It does the work while you do something else.

- Dehydrator; good for preparing crackers and snacks, and for drying fruit, vegetables, nuts, and seeds for later use.

- Juicer (heavy-duty preferred) for increasing the quantity of vitamin- and mineral-boosting fresh vegetables.

Avoid microwaves. We are lucky these days to have abundant labor-saving devices for cooking and cleanup. Most, but not all, provide healthy food quickly. The exception is the microwave oven. Not only does it heat food poorly and unevenly, but it also negatively alters the nutrients in ways conventional heating doesn't (de Pomerai et al. 2003). You can heat up leftovers in just a few minutes in a pot on the stove with a little water, or in the oven or toaster oven in the same glass container in which it was stored. It tastes better, and you don't have to worry about potential harm from consuming plastic or other harmful compounds. Microwaving is still an experiment, and initial results aren't promising.

NECESSARY STAPLES

Ancient peoples dried fruit, vegetables, nuts, seeds, and grains to ensure they had food all year long. You can do the same, but many of these foods can potentially irritate your intestines. Don't have foods around that you are sensitive or allergic to. That way you won't be tempted by foods your body doesn't need or appreciate. Hopefully your whole family will help you with this, especially once they realize your health is at stake. With healthy staple foods on hand, you'll always have something to eat. Staple foods are those that are eaten frequently and store well for extended periods without preservatives or extensive processing. Many store well for months in sealed jars in a cool, dark place, such as your cabinet. You can easily make grains and beans more digestible by soaking and slow cooking. By making a large amount when you slow cook, you can freeze the extra in separate servings to use during the next few weeks. As always, include only foods that work for you. Here are some examples you might try:

- Dried beans—whatever kinds work with your digestive system.

- Whole grains, such as brown rice, basmati rice, millet, buckwheat, amaranth, and quinoa.

- A variety of raw nuts and seeds, such as sunflower seeds, pumpkin seeds, flaxseeds, sesame seeds, walnuts, almonds, cashews, and pecans. Keep them in your refrigerator or freezer to prevent oxidation and stale tastes.

- Dried seaweed. You can use nori sheets to wrap nearly anything and add excellent minerals to your diet. They keep nearly forever in a dry cabinet.

- Sun-dried tomatoes, dried sweet peppers, or both add a wonderful taste of summer to many dishes, plus they contain considerable vitamin C.

- Organic frozen vegetables can be cooked in the steamer or added to soups and stews. They retain nearly as many of their vitamins as fresh vegetables do, and all of the mineral content (Hudson, Dalal, and LaChance 1985).

- Fish, such as sardines, salmon, herring, and albacore tuna, provide good protein and essential fatty acids. Get fresh, flash-frozen, or those packed in spring water or, if you can find it, in extra-virgin olive oil. Avoid fish packed in "pure olive oil," the lowest grade, which is extracted with high heat and solvents.

- Frozen stock; make your own (see chapter 8) and store in freezer jars in your freezer. Freezer jars are slightly thicker than canning jars and have a conical shape that makes it easy to remove the frozen stock. You can get them cheaply by the case at most hardware stores.

- Garlic and ginger keep well in a ventilated garlic jar or a covered basket, which allows some air circulation so the contents don't get moldy.

- Keep onions in your refrigerator. They keep longer, and if cut when cold, they don't cause nearly as many tears as room-temperature onions. Darkness keeps them from sprouting.

- Root vegetables, leeks, cabbage, and winter squash keep in the refrigerator for weeks or even longer. Our ancestors depended on these foods through the long winters.

- Healthy oils such as extra-virgin olive, unrefined coconut, and palm oils are stable for many months in a cool, dark place. Organic clarified butter (ghee) and rendered organic chicken, duck, lamb, or beef fat keep in the freezer for months.

- Cultured vegetables, such as sauerkraut, and cultured dairy, such as yogurt, kefir, and aged cheeses, are traditional ways of preserving foods. They keep for months, and hard cheeses even keep for years. Many are inexpensive and easy to make yourself (see the resources).

- An assortment of herbs and spices. No kitchen is complete without a variety of dried plants to add flavor, color, and interest to your meals. Many are healing to the gut. Consider growing your own herbs in a planter so you always have fresh organic herbs. Experiment by adding one or two herbs or spices to a dish. Add enough to notice its flavor but not so much as to overpower the food. See what works best with your sense of taste. Here are some I keep in my kitchen:

Allspice	Dill	Parsley
Basil	Fennel seed	Sage
Cardamom	Garlic powder	Sea salt (Celtic or Himalayan)
Cinnamon	Ginger	Stevia
Coriander	Mint	Thyme
Curry powder	Oregano	Turmeric

SOAKING, SPROUTING, OR FERMENTING NUTS, SEEDS, BEANS, AND GRAINS FOR OPTIMAL DIGESTION

If you have IBS, you need to make all your foods as easily digestible as possible. Soaking, sprouting, or fermenting nuts, seeds, beans, and grains improves digestion of these nutrient-rich foods. Nuts, seeds, beans, and grains are the beginnings of new plants. When kept damp, with added warmth and light from the sun, they begin to sprout. A seed can wait months, or even years, until these conditions are met. If eaten by an animal and passed through intact, the seed would arrive on the ground with perfect conditions for sprouting and growth, so all plant seeds try to protect themselves from being digested. The hulls and bran of most seeds contain enzyme inhibitors to prevent their digestion, should they be eaten. All nuts, seeds, beans, and grains also contain substances called *phytates*, which bind tightly to minerals so the new plant has what it needs to grow. Though these protective compounds help the seeds, they can prevent us from digesting them and make the many minerals therein unavailable to us. Ancient peoples discovered that soaking, sprouting, or fermenting nuts, seeds, beans, and grains allows us to digest them more easily, and research confirms the reason behind this: that these processes reduce phytates and remove enzyme inhibitors (Fallon and Enig 1999). The results also taste sweeter and, once sprouted, contain more vitamins. If you have had problems digesting these foods in the past, it's worth the extra few minutes to prepare these foods this way.

It's easy to set up your kitchen for soaking, sprouting, and fermenting seeds, nuts, seeds, beans, and grains. All you need is a quart jar, a piece of screen or cloth large enough to cover its top, a rubber band or jar-lid ring, and an out-of-the-way portion of your counter. (See the recipes in chapter 8.)

PREPARING CULTURED FOODS

For good gut health, it's important to include healthful bacteria in your diet on a regular basis. Today many good sources of beneficial bacteria are available (in the form of probiotic preparations); however, some may contain added sweeteners or other ingredients, such as thickeners, that do *not* benefit your gut. It's very easy and inexpensive to make your own cultured foods. No additional equipment is *necessary*, but a few things can make the process much easier. For cultured vegetables, you can use quart-sized mason jars, or for larger quantities, a ceramic crock. A potato masher, wooden pounder, or meat hammer is useful for tamping down the cabbage or other vegetables, and eliminating air.

Many people with IBS are allergic or sensitive to dairy products. Thankfully, you can make many nondairy cultured foods at home, such as vegetable ferments: for example, sauerkraut, sour beets, pickled cucumbers, garlic, ginger and peppers, salsa, and chutney (Katz 2003; Fallon and Enig 1999). Included in the recipe section is a basic recipe for homemade sauerkraut that you can vary to include other vegetables (see chapter 8). Today, when you buy these foods in the grocery, they've usually been prepared with added grain vinegar so that they don't contain any beneficial bacteria. But see the resources for exceptions.

Coconut-water kefir is an excellent nondairy, bacteria-rich beverage that helps replace healthy gut bacteria (Gates 2006). It's very simple to make because it ferments at room temperature. Its sour, effervescent taste resembles a lemon soda, but there's no sugar left after fermentation. A source for the starter kefir grains is listed in the resources.

For those who *can* consume dairy without increasing their IBS symptoms, homemade yogurt fermented for at least twenty-four hours is a good source of healthful bacteria and partially digested protein. The yogurt available in the store has been fermented for only six to eight hours, so it still contains lactose. It takes at least twenty-four hours for healthful bacteria to convert all of the lactose to lactic acid. To make your own yogurt, you need some way to incubate milk with a starter at 100 to 110 degrees Fahrenheit. You can do this in a gas oven that has a pilot light, in a large cooler chest with an electric hot pad, in a dehydrator, or in a yogurt incubator made for this purpose. Our ancestors made cultured foods regularly, as a way to preserve milk before refrigeration was invented and to provide them with good digestive health. Totally fermented yogurt is tart and has no lactose. However, it still contains casein, the protein in dairy products, so you should still avoid it if you have a milk allergy or sensitivity.

Set up your kitchen so you can enjoy the process as well as the final products. A well-stocked kitchen makes food preparation much easier. If you have the tools you need to speed up food preparation, you can enjoy the creative process of preparing foods both you and your family will enjoy. Get the kids involved in food preparation. Cooking is a basic skill everyone needs to learn, but make it fun.

With healthy foods on hand, you'll be less tempted to go out and eat processed foods that can irritate your intestines, plus you'll save money in the long run (on food and doctor's bills). The next chapter shows you how to make menu plans based on the rotation-diet principle, and create a basic shopping list. Getting organized leads to habits that improve efficiency, allowing you more time to express yourself in the kitchen and elsewhere.

7

What Do I Eat?

Many whole food choices are available to help heal your irritable bowel. You may not have tried some of these delicious, nutritious, and easy-to-prepare foods yet, or you may have actually expanded your diet and enjoy the increased variety of foods, despite having to avoid certain foods. Emphasize vegetables, and eat cooked vegetables if diarrhea is your primary IBS symptom. If you tend to have constipation, include more raw vegetables.

Eliminate any foods that prove to be a problem for you, depending on the results of your provocative food testing or allergy-sensitivity testing. Avoiding these problem foods helps you notice an improvement in your digestive health. Many people are allergic or sensitive to gluten (the protein in wheat and other grains), cow's milk and other dairy products, eggs, and soybeans. Eliminating these foods is a good starting place if you can't do the elimination diet or get a food allergy test.

Plan meals for balance and variety. Make grocery lists and menus based on your preferences and digestive capability. Keep staple foods and spices on hand. Each meal should consist of a serving of a protein food, either animal or vegetable, and a wide variety of vegetables. Eat three to four times as many vegetables as protein-rich foods, and be sure to include some healthy fats or oils. Incorporate vegetables into your breakfast, too. Include foods from several colors of the rainbow in each meal or snack. The goal is to choose a protein, a leafy vegetable, and other vegetables for each meal or each day. Keep it simple. You don't need to be a gourmet cook to eat well. A simple and satisfying meal that's easy on the digestive system is steamed vegetables with a baked or roasted meat or fish. Soups are especially fast and easy to prepare. Experiment with individual spices so your foods take on a variety of flavors.

SAMPLE MEALS

An example of a simple, well-balanced meal is five ounces of baked fish, one cup of steamed kale, one-half cup of steamed carrots, one-half cup of sautéed broccoli with mushrooms and garlic, and one cup of green salad with cherry tomatoes, dressed with olive oil and lemon. A snack might be meal leftovers, a handful of nuts or seeds, or a smoothie. Here are some sample meals for four days. You can find the italicized recipes in chapter 8.

Day 1

Breakfast	*Breakfast Patties* on steamed kale, carrots, cauliflower
Snack	*Creamy Cashew Milk*
Lunch	Tuna salad on salad greens, *Guacamole, Baked Corn Chips*
Snack	*Banana-Almond Bread*
Dinner	*Slow-Cooked Turkey Thigh* with carrots, steamed kale, *Mashed Garlic Cauliflower*, and green salad with lemon-garlic dressing
Snack	*Banana-Cashew Pudding*

Day 2

Breakfast	Smoked salmon, steamed spinach, crookneck squash, broccoli
Snack	*Nori Snack Roll*
Lunch	*Sardine Salad* on romaine lettuce, snow peas
Snack	*Berry-Coconut Smoothie*
Dinner	*Baked Fish* (salmon) with beets, steamed spinach, broccoli and romaine salad
Snack	*Blueberry Pie*

Day 3

Breakfast	*Green Eggs*; *Easy, Fresh Salsa*; steamed zucchini; celery sticks
Snack	*Green Smoothie*
Lunch	*Chicken-Vegetable Soup*, *Sweet Cucumber Salad*, sliced tomato
Snack	Almonds, *Toasted Sea Palm*
Dinner	*Chicken Italiano*, spaghetti squash, artichoke, portabella mushrooms, green salad
Snack	*Nutty Porridge* with *Almond Milk*

Day 4

Breakfast	Ground beef sautéed with shiitake mushrooms, leeks, chard
Snack	Pear, pumpkin seeds
Lunch	*Baked Winter Squash* stuffed with *Millet-Amaranth Pilaf*
Snack	*Vegetable Juice*, *Liver Pâté*, *Flaxseed Crackers*
Dinner	*Leek-Beef Burgers*, *Winter Squash Soup*, steamed chard
Snack	*Baked Winter Squash* with *Rose-Hip Spread*

SEASONAL MENUS

As the seasons pass, the earth supplies us with different vegetables and fruits. The temperature variations guide our eating preferences, and the weather promotes the growth and maturation of different vegetables, fruits, nuts, and even seafood. We tend to want warming, heavier foods in the colder winter months and lighter, cooling foods in summertime or whenever the weather's hot. The best guide for *your* seasonal foods is your local farmers market. By shopping at the farmers market, you can meet the people who grow the food, taste some samples, discuss how the food was grown, and even learn how to prepare it.

Here are some suggestions for seasonal, seven-day rotation menus:

SPRING AND SUMMER MENU

| | Protein | Vegetables | | | Unrefined Starches | |
		Greens	Crunchy Vegetables	Salad	Roots	Grains (optional)
Serving	3–5 oz.	1 cup	1/2–1 cup	1 cup	1/2 cup	1/2 cup
Sun	salmon	kale	broccoli	arugula	radish	buckwheat
Mon	turkey	nettles	asparagus	parsley	carrot	quinoa
Tue	pork	beet greens	snow peas	spinach	beet	amaranth
Wed	black beans	dandelion greens	summer squash	lettuce	roasted garlic	millet
Thur	chicken	collard greens	cauliflower	cole slaw	turnip	brown rice
Fri	lamb	mint	artichoke	cilantro	parsnip	teff
Sat	halibut	chard	tomato	cucumber	Jerusalem artichoke	wild rice

FALL AND WINTER MENU

| | Protein | Vegetables | | | Unrefined Starches | |
		Greens	Crunchy Vegetables	Soup	Roots	Grains (optional)
Serving	3–5 oz.	1 cup	1/2–1 cup	1 cup	1/2 cup	1/2 cup
Sun	black beans	beet greens	broccoli	beet soup	garlic	buckwheat
Mon	beef	red kale	celery	onion soup	parsnips	corn
Tue	shellfish	mustard greens	green beans	winter squash soup	Spanish black radish	quinoa
Wed	lamb stew	dandelion	fennel	pea soup	rutabagas	teff
Thur	black cod	chard	seaweed	miso soup	daikon	brown rice
Fri	turkey	collards	Brussels sprouts	cauliflower soup	turnips	amaranth
Sat	chicken	cabbage	artichoke	chicken soup	yam	millet

FOUR-DAY ROTATION PLANNING

The goal of the rotation diet is to ensure that you don't eat the same food more than once every four days, in order to prevent food sensitivities. Choose foods from several categories each day. You may choose several foods from a category, and to maintain balance, be sure to choose at least one protein, three vegetables, one fat, and one booster food each meal.

If you know you are sensitive to a particular food, don't eat it, even if it's listed as a possible food choice. Plenty of other options are available to allow you to avoid that food. Be aware that if you are sensitive to a particular food, you may also be sensitive to its close relatives. For instance, apricots, nectarines, peaches, and plums are all closely related. If you are sensitive to nectarines, you may want to avoid apricots, peaches, and plums for a while, possibly three months. Afterward you may find that your IBS has calmed down enough to test the related foods on their rotation day.

Choose individual foods from the following general categories to provide protein, fat, and carbohydrate in each meal. Each vertical column represents a day on the rotation diet. You don't need to eat everything listed for each day. Just use this list as a guide to help you avoid repeating a food more often than every four days, to reduce possible reactions.

FOUR-DAY ROTATION: Proteins			
Day 1	**Day 2**	**Day 3**	**Day 4**
Cold-water or ocean fish: 3–6 oz.			
Albacore or Yellowfin tuna	Clams	Crab, Soft shell crab	Black sea bass
Butterfish, Black cod, Sable fish	Mussels	Crawfish, Florida lobster	Haddock
Ocean perch	Octopus	Lobster	Hake, Hoki, Pacific whiting
Salmon	Oysters	Shrimp, Prawns	Mahi mahi
Sardines, Herring, Anchovies	Scallops		Pacific halibut, from Alaska
	Squid		

Poultry, organic, including organs: 3–5 oz.			
Chicken	Ostrich	Quail	Duck
Cornish game hen	Turkey	Squab	Goose
Lean meat, organic, including organs: 3–4 oz.			
Beef	Goat	Ham, Bacon	Deer or other Venison
Buffalo	Lamb, Mutton	Pork	Rabbit
Beans or other legumes, soaked, sprouted, or fermented: 1/2 cup			
Azuki, Adzuki, Black turtle beans	Garbanzo, Chickpeas	Lentils	Fava beans (faba)
Mung beans	Pinto beans	Peas, Split peas	Lima beans

FOUR-DAY ROTATION: Vegetables

Day 1	Day 2	Day 3	Day 4
Green leafy vegetables, cooked or raw: 1 cup			
Arugula, Rocket	Celery	Amaranth Greens	Dandelion greens
Bok choy	Cilantro	Beet greens	Endive
Cabbage	Mint	Chard	Lettuce, all kinds
Collard greens	Nettles (cooked)	Lamb's Quarters	Radicchio
Kale, all kinds	Parsley	Spinach	
Mustard greens			
Watercress			
Crunchy vegetables: 1/2 cup			
Broccoli, Broccoli rabe or Rapini	Artichoke	Okra	Cucumber
Brussels sprouts	Asparagus	Peas, Snow peas	Squash, summer and winter, all kinds
Cauliflower	Green beans	Peppers, all kinds	
Kohlrabi		Tomato, Tomatillo	

FOUR-DAY ROTATION: Fats

Day 1	Day 2	Day 3	Day 4
Nuts and seeds, raw, organic: 1–4 tablespoons			
Almond	Flaxseed	Chia seed	Cashew
Brazil nut	Pecan	Hemp seed	Macadamia
Coconut	Sesame seed	Pine nut	Pistachio
Peanut	Walnut	Sunflower seed	Pumpkin seed
Fats and oils, unrefined and organic: 1–3 teaspoons			
Coconut oil	Flax oil (never heat)	Duck fat	Macadamia oil
Palm oil	Sesame oil	Lard, bacon fat	Olive oil

FOUR-DAY ROTATION: Booster Foods

Day 1	Day 2	Day 3	Day 4
Spices and herbs: As desired to add flavor and variety to meals			
Allspice	Basil	Caraway	Cardamom
Cumin	Cilantro Coriander	Cayenne	Chives
Horseradish	Dill	Chili	Cinnamon
Mace	Oregano	Paprika, red pepper	Garlic
Mustard seed	Marjoram	Rosemary	Ginger
Nutmeg	Parsley	Thyme	Turmeric
Sage	Stevia		
Seaweeds, important sources of iodine and trace minerals: 1 tsp			
Arame	Hijiki	Chlorella	Dulse
Spirulina	Nori	Sea palm	Sea lettuce
Mushrooms: 1/2 cup			
Black trumpet	Maitake	Crimini (portabello)	Enoki
Chanterelle	Morel	Shiitake	Porcini
Oyster mushroom	Truffle		

FOUR-DAY ROTATION: Unrefined Starches			
Day 1	**Day 2**	**Day 3**	**Day 4**
Root veggetables: 1/2 cup			
Radish, all kinds	Carrot	Beet	Fennel
Rutabaga (swede)	Celeriac	Jerusalem artichoke	Onion, Garlic, Leek, Shallot
Sweet potato, yam	Celery root		
	Parsnip	Potato	Yucca (cassava)
Turnip			
Grains: 1/4–1/2 cup			
Buckwheat	Brown rice	Amaranth	Millet
Oats (certified gluten free)	Brown Basmati rice	Teff	Wild rice
	Quinoa		

FOUR-DAY ROTATION: Unrefined Sweets			
Day 1	**Day 2**	**Day 3**	**Day 4**
Fruit, preferably fresh: 1 medium whole fruit or 1/2 cup			
Apple	Apricot	Blueberries	Banana
Blackberries	Cherries	Cranberries	Cantaloupe
Pears	Figs	Grapefruit	Mango
Pomegranate	Kiwi	Grapes	Melon (all kinds)
Raspberries	Nectarine	Lemon	Papaya
Rose hips	Peach	Lime	Pineapple
Strawberries	Plums, Prunes	Orange	Watermelon

TIPS FOR EATING OUT

Enlist support. Before going out, ask your dining partner to help you stick to your program. Call the restaurant in advance to let them know what you need and to ensure they can provide it. Many are very willing to accommodate their customers if given a heads-up.

To Avoid Gluten, Dairy, or Other Allergens

■ When the server brings the breadbasket, send it away. If your dining partner insists on keeping the breadbasket, have him or her keep it out of your reach.

■ Tell the waitperson exactly what you need to avoid, specifying wheat, rye, barley, oats, gluten, starch, flour, pasta, couscous, bread, breading, and so on. Not everyone knows what pasta or couscous are made from.

■ Ask questions. Ignorance isn't an excuse for making poor choices! Look at the vegetable options and preparation choices for different dishes, and mix and match to get what you need.

■ Whenever it's available, have the grilled or baked cold-water fish or organic meat. Double-check that the fish or meat is not breaded or fried with other wheat-containing foods.

■ Start with a deep-green leafy salad with olive oil and lemon. Ask that it not include croutons.

■ Skip the starchy carbs usually served, especially if they are refined (for example, mashed potatoes, white rice, pasta), and order double veggies and a salad instead. Ask if they can be prepared very simply, such as sautéed in olive oil, steamed, or roasted.

■ Try new vegetables; this is a great opportunity to get your three servings of vegetables per meal and to sample ones you don't normally cook at home.

■ Support restaurants that provide you with the foods you need. Bring friends with you and refer others to these enlightened places.

To Completely Avoid Gluten, Avoid All of the Following

Alcoholic beverages, including grain alcohol, ale, beer, malt beverages, cordials, liqueurs, gin, vodka, whiskey, bourbon, rye, vermouth, aquavit

Anything breaded or fried with breaded foods

Barley

Barley malt

Bran

Bulgur

Candy (many are dusted with wheat flour)

Canned meat products

Caramel color (sometimes made from malt)

Chewing gum

Communion wafers

Couscous

Cracked wheat

Cracker crumbs

Denture adhesives

Dextrin

Distilled vinegar (white vinegar)

Dried fruit

Durum wheat

Farina

Flavorings and extracts (if they contain alcohol)

Flour (sometimes in ice cream, ketchup, mayonnaise, self-rising cornmeal, and instant coffee)

Frozen turkey (often injected with hydrolyzed vegetable protein)

Gluten flour

Graham flour

Hydrolyzed plant protein (HPP)

Hydrolyzed vegetable protein (HVP)

Imitation cheese

Imitation seafood

Luncheon meat

Malt and its extract

Maltodextrin

Medicines (ask your doctor)

Modified food starch

Oat bran

Oats (unless certified gluten free)

Pasta

Rice syrup (often contains barley malt)

Rye

Semolina

Starch

Thickener

Vegetable gum

Wheat (including berries, flakes, germ, germ oil, starch)

Whole grains

Whole rye

Whole wheat

Remember, wheat free isn't gluten free, and low gluten isn't gluten free. Read all labels thoroughly, or call the manufacturer if you need more information.

CHAPTER 8

Try It, You'll Like It

Unless you try something new, you'll never know how your health can improve. You may find you like vegetables when they are prepared in new and different ways from how you've had them before. You may discover you enjoy cooking for yourself and others, once you have guidelines and easy recipes. Some of the recipes in this chapter are new takes on old favorites. Others are specially formulated to relieve an irritated bowel. All are gluten, dairy, and sugar free.

If you tend to have loose stools or diarrhea as your primary IBS symptom, focus on cooked vegetables and soup recipes, and avoid salads and other cold foods. If you tend to be constipated, include plenty of raw vegetables, salads, and smoothies in your daily diet. Anybody can be allergic or sensitive to anything. If you are sensitive or allergic to any food, try avoiding it completely to allow time for your gut to heal. You'll feel better when you do.

SPECIAL INGREDIENTS

Though some of the ingredients in these recipes differ from what you are used to, they are important to help you deal with IBS. You can find these special ingredients in health food stores or Asian groceries, on the Internet, or at large supermarkets. If you don't find what you need in your local supermarket, ask the manager to order it for you.

Stevia: As mentioned in chapter 5, stevia is a South American herb used for thousands of years that's fifty times sweeter than sugar. Stevia is antifungal, so those with IBS, diabetes, and candidiasis can safely use it. The powdered green leaf tastes better (and is more nutritious) than stevia extracts. To hide any bitter aftertaste, try using less stevia and adding cinnamon or other spices.

Raw Honey: Used since ancient times, raw honey is nearly solid at room temperature. It has never been heated, so the healthy enzymes are still intact. Also, often it's not filtered, so it contains some bee pollen as well. If consumed in small amounts daily, local, unfiltered honey is purported to help desensitize you to local pollens (Ishikawa et al. 2008). Since honey is sweeter than sugar, use it sparingly and only if necessary. Never give raw honey to a child under age one, due to the possible presence of botulism spores, which a baby's system can't deal with, but older children and adults have no problem with. Avoid honey if you have candida.

Coconut Oil: Coconut oil contains medium-chain fatty acids, including *lauric acid*, that aren't stored but can provide energy on the cellular level. Lauric acid is also found in mother's milk, and the body converts it to *monolaurin*, an antiviral, antifungal, and antimicrobial compound that helps strengthen the immune system (Enig 2000). You can cook with coconut oil or add it to any recipe that calls for butter or shortening. The better brands have a fragrance of coconut. One inexpensive brand I tried had a distinct odor of solvents. Soy oil producers popularized the notion that the saturated fat in coconut raises cholesterol, but this has proved to be false (Ibid.).

Coconut Cream Concentrate: Coconut cream concentrate, or coconut butter, is a delightful alternative to chocolate, because it's slightly sweet and feels similar to chocolate in the mouth, but doesn't contain the irritating alkaloids chocolate does. This concentrate is made with coconut oil and finely ground, dried coconut meat. You can also add it to warm water and use it in any recipe as you would coconut milk.

Coconut Water: Coconut water is the slightly sweet fluid contained in young green coconuts (Thai coconuts). Since it's a good source of electrolytes, it's used as a sports drink for rehydration. You can obtain it directly from a fresh coconut (it looks like a white, cone-topped cylinder) at Asian markets or health food stores. Some health food stores have canned or juice-box versions available, but the advantage of the fresh form is that you can also scoop out the delicious, soft, sweet, gelatin-like coconut meat and blend it into your recipe for added fiber.

Flaxseeds: As discussed earlier, flaxseeds soothe the digestive tract in many ways: Their fiber lubricates the bowel and feeds beneficial bacteria. Flax contains 57 percent omega-3 fatty acids, which the body needs to produce healing, anti-inflammatory *prostaglandins* (Enig 2000). Flaxseeds also contain a compound called *lignan*, which has antioxidant properties and helps the liver detoxify excess estrogen (Penttinen-Damdimopoulou et al. 2009). Flax not only benefits the cardiovascular and immune systems and helps heal leaky gut, it also has antimicrobial properties (Wood 1999).

To make sure the omega-3 fatty acids don't oxidize, keep flaxseeds in the refrigerator and grind them in a dry blender or a dedicated coffee grinder just before using. The unbroken hull of the seed helps protect its delicate oils. Never roast flaxseeds, because heat above 250 degrees Fahrenheit and oxygen can damage their essential fatty acids. Storing them in the refrigerator or freezer helps protect them from going rancid for months. They should taste delicately nutty, not bitter or stale.

Flaxseed Oil: Pressed from flaxseeds, flaxseed oil contains the same healing omega-3 fatty acids but little or no beneficial fiber. Use flaxseed oil in salad dressings or as a garnish on cooked foods, but never heat it or cook with it, because it's fragile and oxidizes easily. Keep flaxseed oil in the freezer to preserve freshness and flavor.

Nutritional Yeast: Made specifically for the health food industry, nutritional yeast is similar to brewer's yeast, a by-product of beer-making. Rich in B vitamins and minerals, both are booster foods, helping improve energy and blood sugar regulation. If you are sensitive to yeast or have candidiasis, test your reaction to a small amount before including it regularly in your diet. If you experience bloating or allergic reactions to yeast in general, avoid all forms.

Seaweeds: Seaweeds, or sea vegetables, are full of all the trace minerals so deficient in refined foods. They are used in small amounts in many of these recipes to improve mineral balance and promote healing. The types that can help people with IBS are dulse, nori, wakame, hijiki, and sea palm. Avoid kombu and agar, because they contain too much of a gelatin-like thickener for carbohydrate-sensitive individuals.

Whey: Whey is the liquid portion that's separated from the solid curds in cheese-making. (Remember Little Miss Muffet, eating her curds and whey?) You can purchase whey as a concentrated, dried powder, or you can collect it as a liquid when you drain yogurt through a thin cloth over a bowl. If you aren't allergic to dairy, it's an excellent source of absorbable protein and contains necessary minerals.

BEVERAGES

What we drink is just as important as what we eat. "Dilution is the solution to internal pollution" (Jones 1995, 64). Pure, filtered water is great, but sometimes we want something with flavor. Nutritious beverages are another way to increase your nutrient intake in a fun, tasty, easy-to-absorb way. Be creative.

MORNING CLEANSER

This refreshing alternative to coffee or tea restores your body's pH balance and is very cleansing. Lemon juice flushes out impurities and excess mucus, cleans the liver, and acts as a natural appetite suppressant (Wood 1999). Meyer lemons are a particularly sweet variety. For optimal benefits, wait 15 to 30 minutes before consuming other beverages or foods.

> **1/2 fresh lemon, juiced (about 1 teaspoon to 1 tablespoon of juice)**
>
> **1 cup warm water**
>
> **Pinch of stevia (optional)**

Squeeze the lemon into the warm water. Add the stevia, if desired, and sip slowly.

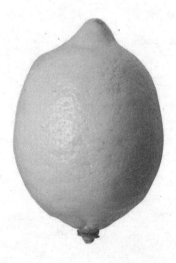

LEMON LIVER FLUSH

You can drink this beverage each morning to detoxify and gently stimulate the liver. Cayenne is warming and increases metabolism, but if you are sensitive to nightshades, replace it with black pepper.

1 organic lemon, juiced

2 cups pure water

1 teaspoon organic extra-virgin olive oil

1/2 teaspoon chopped fresh ginger

Pinch of stevia (optional)

Pinch to 1/8 teaspoon cayenne or black pepper (optional)

Blend all ingredients together and sip slowly.

CHIA FRESCA

This fiber-rich beverage is energy boosting, refreshing, and so simple.

8 ounces coconut water

1/2 lemon, juiced

2 teaspoons chia seeds

Combine all ingredients and let sit for 10 minutes or until the seeds become gel-like. Stir and enjoy.

Makes 1 serving containing 120 calories, 4 grams of protein, 17 grams of carbohydrate, 5 grams of fat, 8 grams of fiber, and 652 milligrams of potassium (19 percent of the recommended daily allowance)

JUICING SUGGESTIONS

Fresh vegetable juices are a great way to consume large quantities of vegetables (and thus increase nutrient intake) without the bulk of so much fiber. A high-quality home juicer is an excellent investment in your health. Bottled juices are pasteurized, which destroys enzymes and some vitamins, and have added chemical preservatives. Making your own fresh vegetable juices optimizes your nutritional benefit. Use nonsweet vegetables instead of fruit, because sweet juices can quickly create blood sugar imbalance and liver metabolism issues. If you are constipated and need more fiber, you may want to use a high-powered blender instead of a juicer (which removes the fiber) to prepare liquefied vegetables with their fiber included, or add 1 tablespoon of ground flaxseeds or chia seeds to your juice.

VEGETABLE JUICE

4 carrots

4 stalks celery

1 beet

1 cup spinach

1 cup fresh parsley

1/2 lemon, juiced

1/2 teaspoon dulse granules (seaweed)

1 teaspoon fresh or dried dill leaf (optional)

1/2 teaspoon garlic powder (optional)

Pinch of cayenne powder (optional)

Juice the vegetables. Squeeze in the lemon juice. Sprinkle in the fresh or dried dulse, dill, garlic powder, or cayenne to taste, and stir.

Makes 1 serving containing 139 calories, 3 grams of protein, 31 grams of carbohydrate, 0 grams of fat, and 0 grams of fiber

NUT MILKS

Lactose, the sugar in dairy milks, triggers major IBS symptoms for many (Nichols and Faass 1999). Homemade nut milks are a delicious nondairy way to deal with a lactose intolerance or milk allergy. Most nuts grow on trees, which have deep roots and can thus accumulate a lot of trace minerals, so nuts are a good source of selenium and other trace minerals as well as vitamin E (good for the heart), and vitamin B6. Vitamin B6 is very deficient in most other foods since heat and light damage it, therefore mostly destroying it in processing (Gyorgy 1954). You can use nut milks in most of the ways you use cow or goat milk. To save money and avoid refined sweeteners, make your own nut milk of your choice. Remember to use a variety of nuts (in rotation) to avoid allergenic reactions.

Soy milk is *not* a good option because so many people with IBS are sensitive to soy. Soybeans contain *phytic acid*, which ties up minerals you need to heal your gut, and compounds called *goitrogens*, which can reduce the effectiveness of your thyroid hormone. Soy also contains compounds that inhibit protein digestion (*trypsin inhibitors*), which can lead to indigestion, IBS, and allergic reactions.

ALMOND MILK

3/4 cup raw, organic almonds

2 cups water

1/4 cup raisins, soaked until soft (optional)

1. Soak the almonds, in enough water to cover them completely, for 8 hours or overnight.

2. Drain the almonds. In a blender, blend together until smooth the almonds, raisins, if desired, and 1 cup of fresh water. Add the second cup of water and blend for another minute.

3. Strain using a fine strainer or thin cloth to remove any solid bits, and refrigerate. You may save the strained almond-raisin meal to add to your breakfast porridge.

Makes about 2 1/2 cups, each 1/2 cup serving containing 134 calories, 4 grams of protein, 9 grams of fat, 12 grams of carbohydrate, and 2 grams of fiber

CREAMY CASHEW MILK

To make cashews edible, their toxic outer shells are roasted and removed, and then an inner shell is removed, also by roasting. The remaining nuts are then sold as raw, even though technically they have been heated. Raw cashews are naturally sweet, so no additional sweeteners are needed.

1 cup organic, raw cashews

3 cups water

1. In a blender, add the cashews and water, and let soak for about 1 hour.

2. Blend the nuts and water together until totally blended. Strain the milk to remove any larger pieces.

Makes about 3 1/2 cups, each 1/2 cup serving containing 131 calories, 4 grams of protein, 10 grams of fat, 7 grams of carbohydrate, and 1 gram of fiber

CASHEW-FLAXSEED MILK

Everyone I know who has tried this cashew milk has raved about it. The flax-seeds thicken the milk and add essential fatty acids.

1/2 cup raw cashews

3 cups water

1 tablespoon flaxseeds, finely ground

In a dry blender, grind the cashews to a fine powder. While blending, add the water slowly; then add the ground flaxseeds. Blend together well, and strain (if desired).

Makes about 3 cups, each 3/4 cup serving containing 88 calories, 3 grams of protein, 7 grams of fat, 5 grams of carbohydrate, and 1 gram of fiber

SMOOTHIES

A smoothie makes a satisfying snack or meal. Quick to make, smoothies are also a good way to incorporate booster foods into your diet. You can use just about any fruit or vegetable in a smoothie. Use whole fruit instead of fruit juices, since the fiber in whole fruit is necessary to regulate blood sugar. Don't add ice to your smoothies, since cold foods reduce digestive function (Drettner 1964), and remember to sip smoothies slowly for optimal digestion and nutrient absorption.

BERRY-COCONUT SMOOTHIE

This meal in a glass is good anytime, especially in the morning, since it provides the protein needed to jump-start metabolism. Use all organic ingredients for a higher nutrient content and better taste, and to prevent pesticide exposure. If you aren't sensitive to dairy, you can substitute whey protein for the rice or hemp protein. Experiment with various seasonal fruits and even vegetables for a variety of flavors and nutrients.

1 cup fresh seasonal fruit (strawberry, blackberry, blueberry, nectarine, peach, plum, mango, or kiwi)

1 cup coconut milk or coconut water

1/2 cup water

2 tablespoons rice protein powder or hemp protein powder

1 to 2 tablespoons ground flaxseeds

1 teaspoon to 1 tablespoon chlorella or spirulina powder

1 teaspoon nutritional yeast or brewer's yeast (optional)

Pinch or more of stevia green-leaf powder (optional)

Put all ingredients into a blender and process at high speed for 3 minutes or until completely smooth. Pour into a tall glass and sip with a straw.

Makes 1 serving containing 435 calories, 21 grams of protein, 31 grams of carbohydrate, 29 grams of fat, and 6 grams of fiber

FRUIT SMOOTHIE

This is a refreshing, cleansing smoothie for those who can eat fresh fruit and the sugars therein.

1 cup fresh organic fruit (pineapple, grapefruit, orange, kiwi, mango, papaya, peach, or plum)

1 banana

1/2 lemon, juiced

1 tablespoon ground flaxseeds

1 to 2 teaspoons nutritional yeast or brewer's yeast

Add all ingredients to a blender and blend until completely smooth, about 3 minutes.

Makes 1 serving containing 231 calories, 52 grams of carbohydrate, 4 grams of fat, 3 grams of protein, and 6 grams of fiber, and providing nearly 100 percent of the recommended daily allowance of vitamin C (90 milligrams)

GREEN SMOOTHIE

This can be thick, like a pudding, or thinned with water to make it more pourable. The fiber from the flaxseeds, chia seeds, or psyllium helps soothe the intestines.

10 to 12 ounces coconut water, or 1 ounce applesauce diluted in 8 ounces water

1/2 avocado

1/2 organic lemon, including rind, seeded

1/2 to 1 cup fresh cilantro or parsley leaves

1 tablespoon ground flaxseeds, chia seeds, or psyllium hulls

1/8 to 1/4 teaspoon stevia

Blend all ingredients in a blender until smooth.

Makes 1 serving containing 243 calories, 27 grams of carbohydrate, 15 grams of fat, 7 grams of protein, and 12 grams of fiber

ENERGY SMOOTHIE

Green powders are very alkalinizing, because of the minerals they contain. They help balance a diet high in animal protein, which can acidify the body. Some brands contain wheatgrass or barley grass juice, which may have gluten. Use pure chlorella or spirulina to avoid gluten.

> **1 banana**
>
> **1 cup strawberries or other berries, fresh or frozen**
>
> **2 tablespoons rice protein powder or hemp protein powder**
>
> **1 teaspoon lecithin**
>
> **1 teaspoon nutritional yeast or brewer's yeast (optional)**
>
> **1/2 to 2 teaspoons chlorella, spirulina, or other green powder**
>
> **1/2 cup nut milk of choice (pages 94 and 95), or coconut water**

In a blender add the fruit, powders, and nut milk or coconut water. Blend on high, adding more liquid, if needed, to mix thoroughly.

Makes 1 serving containing 228 calories, 20 grams of protein, 6 grams of fat, 44 grams of carbohydrate, and 8 grams of fiber

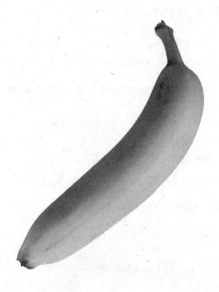

BREAKFAST

Studies show that people who eat breakfast have higher nutrient levels, improved digestion, better control of blood sugar and cholesterol, and decreased risk of heart attack (Affenito 2007). However, many commonly eaten breakfast foods can further irritate the sensitive bowel. These recipes provide alternatives to boxed cereals, pancakes, waffles, doughnuts, and bacon, which are often some of the problem breakfast foods.

Think outside the box. You can eat any healthy food for breakfast. Cold cereal is one of the worst things you can eat for breakfast (or anytime, for that matter) if you have IBS. Research in 1960 at the University of Michigan showed that rats fed the box the cereal came in, along with water and vitamins, lived longer than rats fed the cereal, water, and vitamins (Fallon and Enig 1999). In addition, the usual American breakfast of boxed cereal and milk contains the two most difficult-to-digest compounds, gluten and casein, respectively. Eating any hard-to-digest food for breakfast is a common cause of gas and bloating later in the day. Aim to get at least 25 percent of your daily calories at breakfast, with around 25 percent of your breakfast calories coming from protein.

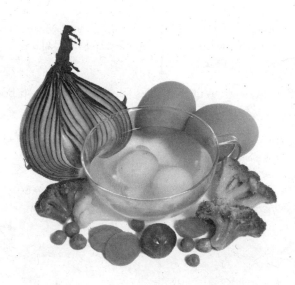

PERFECT SOFT- OR HARD-BOILED EGGS

Eggs are considered the perfect protein food, especially when cooked properly, and the yolk is the most nutrient rich portion. Eggs are good sources of essential fatty acids, vitamins A and D (if hens were pasture raised), and lecithin, which emulsifies cholesterol. However, avoid raw egg white, which contains *avidin*, a compound that binds with *biotin* (an important B vitamin), making biotin unavailable to the body. The perfect soft-boiled egg has a solidly cooked white and a still-liquid yolk. If you dislike runny yolks, cook your eggs a few minutes longer, until the yolks are to your liking. Some people use eggcups to serve soft-boiled eggs. If you don't have eggcups, serve eggs in a small bowl, cracking them in half and scooping them out with a teaspoon. Serve with steamed greens and other vegetables. Submerge hard-boiled eggs in very cold water immediately after cooking for easier peeling.

This technique for cooking eggs ensures they aren't overcooked, to optimize protein digestion and nutrient absorption. Follow these easy steps to enjoy perfect eggs every time.

2 or 3 large organic or pasture-raised eggs

1. Take the eggs out of the refrigerator and allow them to warm to room temperature.

2. Fill a saucepan, large enough to fit all the eggs, with enough water to submerge them completely. Cover the saucepan and bring the water (without the eggs) to a full boil.

3. Gently spoon the eggs into the pan of boiling water. Make sure the eggs are completely covered with water. When the water boils again, cover them and remove them from heat.

4. Allow the eggs to sit in the hot water for 6 minutes for soft-boiled eggs, or 12 minutes for hard-boiled eggs.

5. Remove the eggs from the water and serve. Submerge hard-boiled eggs in ice water for easier peeling.

Makes 1 serving, with two eggs containing 155 calories, 13 grams of protein, 11 grams of fat, 1 gram of carbohydrate, and 0 grams of fiber

POACHED EGGS FLORENTINO

This is another way to get greens into your breakfast.

1 corn tortilla

2 pasture-raised or organic eggs

1 cup (1 ounce) spinach or kale, steamed

1 teaspoon flaxseed oil or 2 teaspoons freshly ground flaxseeds

1. In a shallow saucepan, bring water (about 1-inch deep) to a low boil.

2. Warm the tortilla by putting it in a low-temperature (under 200°F) oven for 10 minutes. Gently break the eggs into the boiling water, without breaking the yolk. Allow them to cook for 2 to 3 minutes, until the egg white is completely opaque. Cook 1 minute longer if you desire a semisolid yolk.

3. Layer the steamed greens onto the tortilla and add the flaxseed oil or flaxseeds.

4. With a slotted spoon, remove the eggs from the water and place them on top of the greens. Serve immediately.

Makes 1 serving containing 241 calories, 15 grams of protein, 15 grams of fat, 13 grams of carbohydrate, and 2 grams of fiber

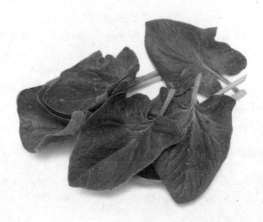

GREEN EGGS

For children or adults, this is a good way to get greens into breakfast. Greens are high in chlorophyll, bioflavonoids, fiber, and minerals, including magnesium, calcium, and potassium. Greens help the liver remove toxins from the body, as well as help improve energy, digestion, and elimination. The beta-carotene they contain specifically helps the intestines (feeding the cells lining them), the immune system (fighting cold and flu), the skin (reducing acne and eczema), and the eyes (improving vision) (Davis 1970). Greens are a major source of minerals, especially magnesium and calcium, for calm nerves, restful sleep, and strong bones. The vitamin D in pasture-raised eggs improves the body's ability to properly absorb and use calcium. We need magnesium to prevent fatigue, mental confusion, irritability, weakness, muscle cramps, asthma, insomnia, stress, heart disease, diabetes, gout, and kidney stones (Murray 1996).

4 to 6 large eggs (organic or pasture raised)

1 to 2 cups organic, raw greens (kale, parsley, cilantro, watercress, spinach, chard, dandelion, or collards)

2 to 3 cloves of garlic or 1/2 teaspoon garlic powder

1 teaspoon dulse granules (seaweed)

1 tablespoon extra-virgin olive oil, or water (optional)

Salsa or tomato slices for garnish

1. Break the eggs into a blender. Add the raw greens, garlic, and dulse, and blend thoroughly until smooth. Add a tablespoon of water or olive oil, if necessary, to blend the greens completely.

2. Heat a skillet to medium with the oil and add the egg-greens mixture. Cook until the eggs are done, either by stirring (scramble style) or by turning down heat, covering, and letting them steam (omelet style) for about 10 to 15 minutes. Alternatively, if using a cast-iron skillet, you can finish cooking them in the oven at 300°F for 15 minutes. When done, the surface will look dry and spring back slowly when depressed, or a fork will come out clean. The dish will still have a beautiful green color.

3. Garnish with salsa or tomato slices, and serve hot.

Serves 2 adults or 4 children, each adult size serving containing 230 calories, 14 grams of protein, 17 grams of fat, 6 grams of carbohydrate, and 1 gram of fiber

BREAKFAST PATTIES

Many of the sausages and breakfast patties on the market have ingredients that are unhealthy for people with IBS, including artificial and "natural" flavorings, coloring, nitrates and nitrites, sugar, fillers, starches, and gums to increase profit margins, and often nonfat dry milk powder to cheaply increase protein content. Consider making your own breakfast sausage patties and individually freezing them for future use.

1 pound ground organic chicken or turkey

1 onion, finely diced

1/4 to 1/2 cup extra-virgin olive oil

2 teaspoons dried sage powder

2 teaspoons dried or fresh oregano

1 teaspoon dried or fresh thyme

2 cloves garlic, minced, or 1 teaspoon garlic powder

2 teaspoons dulse (seaweed)

1/2 to 1 teaspoon salt

1/4 teaspoon ground pepper (optional)

1. Thoroughly mix the ground meat, diced onion, olive oil, and spices in a large bowl with your clean hands, or in a food processor. Add enough olive oil to help achieve adequate moistness, since ground poultry is too dry otherwise.

2. Divide the mixture into 6 equal parts, and roll each part into a ball and flatten it into a patty. The patties will shrink when cooked, so make them about 25 percent larger than you want the cooked patties to be.

3. *To freeze for later use:* Put each patty between layers of waxed paper or into its own bag, and then put 2 or 3 of them into a ziplock bag (which can be reused). Try to eliminate air in the bag to prevent freezer burn.

4. *To cook:* Melt some fat, such as *schmaltz* (chicken fat), or use olive oil in a cast-iron skillet (with a lid to prevent burning) at medium heat. Sauté patties for about 7 minutes on each side (longer if frozen), until golden brown. Serve hot over cooked green leafy vegetables.

Makes four large (1/4 pound) patties, each containing 344 calories, 20 grams of protein, 27 grams of fat, 4 grams of carbohydrate, and 1 gram of fiber

GOLDEN CARROT PANCAKES

This is a great way to have protein-rich but gluten-free pancakes for breakfast or brunch.

> **4 eggs**
>
> **1 cup cooked carrots, or if you have a high-powered blender, 1 large raw carrot**
>
> **1 tablespoon extra-virgin olive or sesame oil**
>
> **1/2 teaspoon cinnamon powder**
>
> **1/2 tablespoon coconut oil**
>
> **Almond or sesame butter, or applesauce**

1. In a blender, add the eggs, carrots, olive or sesame oil, and cinnamon, and blend on high until smooth.

2. Heat a large cast-iron skillet to medium, and add the coconut oil to coat it. Pour the egg-carrot mixture into the pan and cook until the pancake begins to look dry on top. The top should spring back when depressed, or a fork should come out clean.

3. Cut the pancake into quarters and put two quarters on each plate. Spread with almond or sesame butter or applesauce and enjoy.

Makes 2 servings, each consisting of half of one large (9-inch) pancake, containing 229 calories, 13 grams of protein, 17 grams of fat, 7 grams of carbohydrate, and 2 grams of fiber

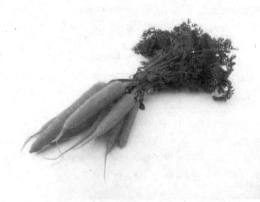

FLAXSEED PUDDING

This is a great way to soothe the intestines. It makes a good addition to breakfast, or you can eat it anytime. For a creamier variation, add ground almonds or pumpkin seeds in addition to the flaxseeds. Add mashed banana or applesauce for a sweeter version.

2 tablespoons organic flaxseeds

1/2 cup hot water

1/4 teaspoon cinnamon or other spice, such as cardamom, coriander, nutmeg, or ginger

1/4 to 1/8 teaspoon green-leaf stevia

1. In a dry blender or a clean coffee grinder, finely grind the flaxseeds.

2. Pour the hot water into a small bowl. Add the spices and stevia to the hot water.

3. Slowly add the ground flaxseeds, allowing them to settle into the water. Mix the seeds into the water-spice mixture until it reaches a pudding-like consistency. Add more hot water if needed.

Makes 1 serving containing 74 calories, 1 gram of protein, 3 grams of fat, 2 grams of carbohydrate, and 2 grams of fiber

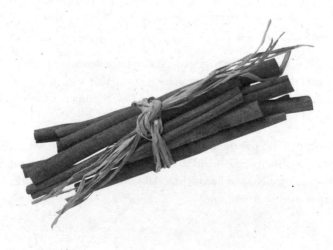

PORRIDGE

Soaking, fermenting, or sprouting all grains, beans, nuts, and seeds helps eliminate or reduce phytates, removes enzyme inhibitors, and even helps break down proteins, making whole grains and beans easier to digest. According to Sally Fallon and Mary Enig in their cookbook *Nourishing Traditions*, "A diet high in unfermented whole grains may lead to serious mineral deficiency and bone loss" (Fallon and Enig 1999, 452). Ancient peoples always fermented or soaked grains and beans before eating them. It takes a bit of preplanning, but when soaked for 8 to 12 hours or overnight with an added acidifier (discussed next), grains begin to taste sweeter as ever-present lactobacillus bacteria convert the starches to sugars. Try this hearty dish for a comforting breakfast. Use any gluten-free grain. If you aren't dairy sensitive, you can use whey liquid as an acidic starter. With longer fermenting times (more than 12 hours in warm weather), the porridge will begin to smell and taste deliciously sour. The acidic apple cider vinegar, lemon juice, or whey kills off any fungus spores and harmful bacteria, and helps the beneficial bacteria ferment the grains. The mixture may get a bit bubbly as it ferments.

1/2 cup gluten-free grain (rice, buckwheat, amaranth, quinoa, millet, teff, certified gluten-free rolled oats, or coarse cornmeal)

1 cup water

1 teaspoon apple cider vinegar or lemon juice (acidic starter)

1. In a medium saucepan, combine the grain, water, and acidic starter. Cover and let soak at room temperature for at least 8 hours (overnight) or up to 24 hours.

2. Heat the saucepan to low to medium. Cook the fermented grain while stirring until thick, about 2 to 3 minutes. Or you may soak the grain in a slow cooker (without heat) and then turn it on low, stirring occasionally until it's thick and warm.

Serve warm with ground flaxseeds and 1 teaspoon of coconut cream concentrate or Nut Milk (pages 94 and 95). You may also wish to add dried coconut meat, Soaked, Dried Nuts or Seeds (page 110), Rose-Hip Spread (page 114), or a sprinkle of stevia green-leaf powder.

NUTTY PORRIDGE

This fermented and slow-cooked cereal, mixed with nuts and seeds, can keep you warm all morning.

2/3 cup whole grain (brown rice, amaranth, millet, quinoa, buckwheat, or coarse cornmeal)

16 (2/3 ounce) organic raw almonds, walnuts, or other raw nuts

2 tablespoons (2/3 ounce) pumpkin seeds (hulled)

2 tablespoons (2/3 ounce) sunflower seeds (hulled)

2 cups water

1 teaspoon lemon juice or apple cider vinegar

1 teaspoon bee pollen

4 teaspoons flaxseed meal or 2 teaspoons flaxseed oil

2 tablespoons Rose-Hip Spread (page 114)

1. Mix the grain, nuts, seeds, water, and lemon juice or vinegar in a small saucepan. Cover and let it sit at room temperature for 8 hours or overnight. Bubbles may form.

2. Put the saucepan on medium-high heat and stir until the cereal thickens, about 1 to 3 minutes.

3. Spoon the porridge into 2 bowls. Divide the bee pollen, flaxseed meal, and Rose-Hip Spread evenly over both servings.

Variation: Use stock instead of water and omit the bee pollen for a savory side dish.

Makes 2 servings, each containing 346 calories, 11 grams of protein, 17 grams of fat, 42 grams of carbohydrate, and 7 grams of fiber

SPROUTING MADE EASY

Sprouting is another way to make grains, seeds, and beans more digestible by removing enzyme inhibitors and phytates, the latter of which interfere with mineral absorption during digestion. In olden days, all grains were either soaked, sprouted, or fermented, which removes the phytates and increases digestibility. Sprouting increases B vitamins and carotenes, and as the leaves form, the little growing plant creates vitamin C.

You can sprout any whole grain, but at least slightly cook grain and bean sprouts before eating them to improve digestibility. Try buckwheat, quinoa, amaranth, millet, or certified gluten-free whole oats (rolled oats won't sprout). Grains will sprout as long as they haven't been broken or irradiated. It's very difficult to sprout rice and teff, so soaking or fermenting them is a better way to prepare them.

After three to six days, you should see both root and leaf parts beginning to grow, and the sprouts are ready to eat. When they are done, you can eat them at once or store them in the refrigerator in their sprouting jar. Just put a lid on the jar, or transfer them to a dry, closed container. Keeping them in a glass jar in the refrigerator reminds you to eat them when you see them. In an opaque container, they can easily be forgotten. Eat seed sprouts on salads, on soups or stews, or by themselves. You can also lightly steam them for 2 minutes, although they will lose some of their nutrients in the cooking process.

Avoid eating large amounts of alfalfa sprouts, because they contain an amino acid called canavanine, an analog of the amino acid arginine, which can interfere with protein synthesis and the immune system and contribute to lupus and other inflammatory conditions (Fallon and Enig 1999). Only young alfalfa sprouts contain canavanine, not the mature plants, so alfalfa herb in tea or as a dried powder is okay.

Here are some good types of beans and seeds to sprout:

- Mung beans—good for the liver; cooling

- Chickpeas (garbanzo beans)—rich in the trace mineral molybdenum, which helps detoxify sulfites

- Broccoli seeds—contain indoles, which help the liver and prevent cancer

- Sunflower seeds—contain vitamin E, essential fatty acids; and minerals

- Pumpkin seeds—contain zinc and essential fatty acids, help eliminate worms

- Onion seeds—spicy and antimicrobial; help the liver detoxify

- Chia seeds—contain vitamin C and soluble fiber (not just to make chia pets)

1/8 cup or less of dry raw beans or seeds

1. Add the beans or seeds to a quart jar. If you use more, the jar will get too full as the sprouts grow. Fill the jar with water and cover with a thin, clean piece of cloth. You can use a rubber band to hold the cloth over the top of the jar.

2. Let the beans or seeds soak overnight or at least 8 hours.

3. The next morning, drain off the water. You don't need to remove the cloth; just pour the water out through the cloth. Let the beans or seeds drain for a few minutes and set the jar at an angle on the counter, out of the way.

4. Rinse and drain the sprouts 3 times a day.

5. After three to six days, the sprouts should have visible roots and stems with small leaves. Store the sprouts in a dry jar for up to one week. If mold forms, throw them out, clean all equipment thoroughly, and begin again.

SNACKS

If you get hungry between meals, it's important to have healthy snacks around to prevent you from grabbing foods that trigger IBS symptoms. Here are a few ideas.

SOAKED, DRIED NUTS OR SEEDS

Raw nuts and seeds are very nutritious and satisfying, plus a good source of vitamins, including B6, as well as minerals and essential fatty acids. Unfortunately, roasting nuts damages these important nutrients. Soaking and redrying them improves digestibility and preserves the vitamins and essential fats. One handful is approximately a one-ounce serving and makes a filling and portable snack.

To prepare the nuts or seeds, you will need a large jar with a lid; a colander or strainer; paper towels or cotton cloths to line whatever you will be drying the nuts or seeds on, such as a baking pan, cookie sheet, or flat baskets like the kind used to support paper plates; and a dehydrator or an oven that can maintain 100 to 118°F. A gas oven with the pilot light on will usually work fine. A 100-watt lightbulb in an electric oven may work too. Check the temperature with an oven thermometer. If the temperature stays below 150°F, the nuts will dry without damaging their essential fatty acids. A warm, sunny place where the nuts won't be disturbed will also work.

2 cups raw seeds or nuts (pumpkin seeds, sunflower seeds, almonds, walnuts, pecans, or hazelnuts)

Filtered water

1 teaspoon unrefined salt (Real Salt, Celtic salt, and Lima salt are the best types. Avoid commercial salt, which contains dextrose, silica, and aluminum. Read the ingredient label.)

1. Place the seeds or nuts in the quart jar. Add the filtered water, filling the jar almost to the top. Add the salt. Put the lid on the jar and shake or stir it a few times to dissolve the salt in the water.

2. Let the nuts soak at room temperature overnight or for 7 to 24 hours.

3. Lay one or two layers of paper towel or cotton cloth over the baking pan, cookie sheet, or flat baskets. Drain the nuts in a colander or strainer, and spread them out over the paper towel. Place the nuts or seeds in the warm oven (100 to 118°F) or dehydrator and let them dry. You may want to stir them around occasionally to speed drying.

4. When completely dry, the nuts will be crunchy, not rubbery. Depending on the humidity, this may take around 24 to 36 hours.

5. Store the nuts or seeds in a glass jar in the refrigerator to keep them fresh.

Makes 8 to 10 servings, with 1 ounce of pecans (20 halves) containing 195 calories, 3 grams of protein, 20 grams of fat, 4 grams of carbohydrate, and 3 grams of fiber

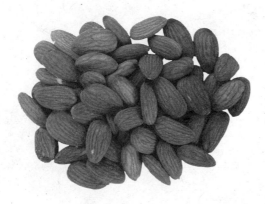

FLAXSEED CRACKERS

If you're gluten sensitive, this is a great substitute for crackers. Incredibly simple to prepare and requiring minimal tools, these special crackers are crunchy and have lots of antioxidants, fiber, and omega-3 fatty acids. Try them with nut butters, Rose-Hip Spread (page 114), smoked salmon, Liver Pâté (page 122), or by themselves.

You'll need an oven (or a dehydrator) that can maintain a temperature of 110 to 118°F. (Don't heat these crackers above 150°F, because they will brown and develop a bitter taste, indicating oxidation.)

For interesting variations, combine blended tomato, red pepper, oregano, and garlic in addition to, or instead of, the blended onion. Add curry spice or cayenne for a spicy cracker. Use ginger, cinnamon, and soaked dried fruit to make a healthy and sweet flaxseed cookie that's full of fiber and low in sugars.

You'll need a blender or food processor, parchment paper (wax paper won't work because it will stick), and a shallow 10 x 15-inch baking tray.

1 cup whole flaxseeds

1 cup water

1 large onion

1/2 teaspoon mineral salt

1. In a medium bowl, soak the flaxseeds in the water until the water is totally absorbed, about 30 minutes. The seeds will be slippery.

2. Purée the onion in the blender or food processor. (It should reduce to about 1 cup.) Add the salt, pulsing the blender to dissolve the salt into the onion mash.

3. Pour the onion mash into the bowl of soaked flaxseeds and stir until mixed.

4. Cover the baking tray with the parchment paper, allowing some of the paper to come up over the sides of the tray. Pour the flax-onion mixture onto the parchment and spread it evenly over the entire tray. It should be about 3/8 inch thick. The crackers will become thinner by half as they dry.

5. Put the pan in the oven for 24 to 36 hours or until the mixture becomes crisp. After about 4 to 6 hours, you can score into individual crackers with a knife or spatula to make them easy to break apart. If it's inconvenient to score them, don't worry, because they still taste fine if broken into uneven pieces. If you find that your oven hasn't sufficiently dried the underside of the crackers, turn them over onto a new parchment and return them to the oven.

6. Once they are completely dry, store the crackers in wax paper in a cool, dry place.

Makes 24 two-inch square crackers, each containing 40 calories, 1 gram of protein, 3 grams of fat, 3 grams of carbohydrate, and 2 grams of fiber

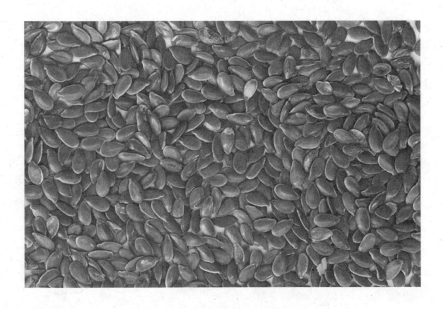

ROSE-HIP SPREAD

Rose hips are the fruit of the rose, and 10 grams of dried rose hips provides 170 to 200 milligrams of vitamin C and antioxidant bioflavonoids. They also contain appreciable amounts of the soluble fiber pectin, which improves bowel health and helps remove toxins. Rose-hip marmalade is a favorite in northern Europe, but this recipe doesn't contain the sugar that marmalades do. Purchase dried, cut, and seeded rose hips from the bulk herbal section of your local health food store or herb supplier. Enjoy the tart taste of this spread as a substitute for jam or jelly. Try a tablespoon of it mixed with porridge. It's not very sweet, especially compared to commercial preserves, but it contains far more nutrition. For a sweeter taste, add 1/4 to 1/2 teaspoon of stevia green-leaf powder or 1 teaspoon of raw honey. You may also add cinnamon, ginger, or other powdered spices to vary the taste. Experiment and enjoy.

1 cup dried and seeded rose hips

2 cups water

2 tablespoons fresh lemon juice

1. Sort through the rose hips to remove any residual seeds and stems.

2. Fill a wide-mouth pint jar halfway with the cleaned rose hips, and cover them with enough pure water to fill the jar. Add the lemon juice. Close the jar lid and shake gently to wet the rose hips.

3. Place the covered jar in the refrigerator for 3 hours, until all the water is absorbed and the rose hips are moist and soft, not crunchy.

4. *Alternate version:* For a smooth, sauce-style version, blend the soaked rose hips thoroughly in a blender.

5. Store in the refrigerator for up to two weeks.

Makes about 1 pint, each tablespoon containing approximately 23 calories, 5 grams of carbohydrate, 3.4 grams of fiber, and 60 milligrams of vitamin C (two-thirds of the recommended daily allowance)

FABULOUS FLAXSEED AND PUMPKIN SEED SPREAD

This is a highly nutritious and satisfying substitute for peanut butter. The essential fatty acid ratio of this spread is 1 to 1.3 omega-3 to omega-6, making it nearly perfect for supporting digestion, reducing inflammation, and maintaining health.

1 cup flaxseeds

1 cup raw pumpkin seeds

1/2 to 3/4 cup olive oil

1/8 teaspoon mineral salt

1. Grind the flaxseeds and pumpkin seeds in a dry blender until very fine. Slowly add the olive oil and continue blending until a thick paste is formed. Add the salt and continue blending thoroughly.

2. Transfer to a wide-mouth jar and store in the refrigerator.

3. Serve on apple slices or crackers, add to cooked cereal, or use as a topping for baked squash or yams.

Makes about 12 servings, each 2 tablespoon serving containing 174 calories, 4 grams of protein, 16 grams of fat, 5 grams of carbohydrate, and 3 grams of fiber

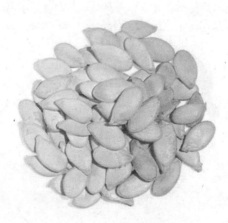

SESAME SEED CHEESE

I discovered this recipe by accident, when I made sesame cream with soaked seeds that was left out on the counter. Four days later, I had this natural non-dairy alternative to cream cheese. Enjoy this cheese's sour tang and appreciate its healthful bacteria.

1 cup hulled sesame seeds

1 1/2 cups pure water

Juice of 1 lemon

1. In a glass quart jar, soak the sesame seeds in the water. Add the lemon juice and let the mixture sit overnight covered in the jar. Don't seal the jar, because the fermentation process needs to "breathe." By the next day, the seeds should have absorbed most of the water, and may be a bit bubbly.

2. Pour off the water, saving it. Put the remaining seeds into a blender or food processor, and blend until creamy. You may need to add a tablespoon or two of the saved water to help get a thick, creamy consistency.

3. Return the blended sesame cream to the jar. Cover it loosely with the jar lid and put it in a cool place with good ventilation for 1 to 4 days. When it's done, it should smell sour, a bit like cheese. If mold grows on the top, skim it off and discard it. Refrigerate the mixture to stop the fermentation once it's at your preferred level of sourness. Serve on Flaxseed Crackers (page 112) or carrot and celery sticks.

Makes approximately 1 pint, each tablespoon containing approximately 80 calories, 2.5 grams of protein, 6 grams of fat, 3.5 grams of carbohydrate, and 2.5 grams of fiber

NORI SNACK ROLL

Here's a yummy way to enjoy sea vegetables. Fill your sushi-like roll with whatever vegetable, fruit, or nut butter you wish; the following filling is just one example. Nori sheets are available at Asian markets and health food stores.

1 sheet nori seaweed (used to make sushi rolls)

1 to 2 tablespoons of nut butter (almond, cashew, or sunflower butter) or tahini

1 to 2 teaspoons coconut cream concentrate (from www .tropicaltraditions.com) or unsweetened shredded coconut

1/4 to 1/3 carrot, cut into long, thin strips with a vegetable peeler

Water to seal the roll

1. Lay the sheet of nori on a cutting board or clean work surface. Spread the nut butter on one third to one half of the nori sheet, across the bottom edge.

2. Spread the coconut cream concentrate or shredded coconut on top of the nut butter.

3. Layer the carrot strips on top of the nut butter–coconut stuffing.

4. Roll the nori sheet over the stuffing. Seal the roll by wetting the edge of the nori sheet with a little water and pressing it to itself as you roll.

5. With a serrated knife, cut the roll into bite-sized sections, or leave it long, like a hand roll, and enjoy.

Each roll is 1 serving containing 205 calories, 5 grams of protein, 18 grams of fat, 10 grams of carbohydrate, and 1 gram of fiber

TOASTED SEA PALM

A healthy replacement for chips, this salty snack food has loads of trace minerals and even some essential fatty acids and proteins, without any harmful trans fats. It's an especially good snack mixed with Soaked, Dried Nuts or Seeds (page 110). You can also grind sea palm and use it on any food instead of salt as a balanced source of minerals. You can get sea palm at health food stores or online.

3 to 4 ounces sea palm

1. Put sea palm pieces on a flat baking dish and toast for 10 minutes in a 250°F oven, until crunchy.

2. Store them in an airtight jar. If they get moist or chewy again, just retoast them as needed.

BAKED CORN CHIPS

You will be amazed at the light, fresh taste of these baked corn chips. Making your own chips can also prevent overconsumption of what should be only an occasional food, and help you completely avoid harmful hydrogenated or refined fats found in store-bought chips.

4 organic, gluten-free corn tortillas

Olive oil

1. Preheat the oven to 350°F.

2. Cut tortillas into 6 to 8 wedges each.

3. Lightly oil a baking pan with olive oil to prevent sticking. Arrange the chips in one layer on the baking pan. Bake for 10 to 15 minutes, until the edges just begin to turn crisp. Don't overcook.

4. Place the chips in a bowl while they're still warm, and serve them with Easy, Fresh Salsa (recipe follows).

Serves 2, each 16-chip serving containing 105 calories, 3 grams of protein, 1 gram of fat, 21 grams of carbohydrate, and 3 grams of fiber

EASY, FRESH SALSA

This salsa is so much tastier and better for you than packaged ones since vitamin C levels are higher in fresh foods than in bottled or packaged ones (Ball 2006). If you're sensitive to peppers, skip the cayenne. Eat this salsa fresh or allow it to marinate for 6 or more hours till the flavor develops. Traditional salsa is allowed to ferment, as sauerkraut is. Use this salsa to make your own delicious guacamole (recipe follows).

3 ripe tomatoes, diced (about one pound)

1 small onion, diced

2 cloves garlic, minced

1/4 to 1/2 cup fresh cilantro, finely chopped

1 tablespoon fresh lemon or lime juice

Pinch cayenne pepper (optional)

Chop all ingredients and mix together in a medium bowl. Serve and enjoy.

Makes 3 servings, each 1/2-cup serving containing 36 calories, 2 grams of protein, 0 grams of fat, 8 grams of carbohydrates, and 2 grams of fiber

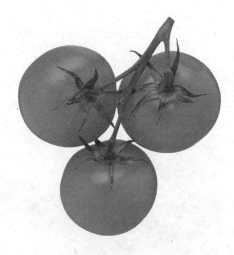

GUACAMOLE

This guacamole is easy to make, especially if you have the Easy, Fresh Salsa (previous recipe) available. If you use a bottled salsa, pick one that's organic and read all the ingredients to avoid added sugar or preservatives.

1 large or 2 medium soft, ripe avocados, about 10 ounces

1 tablespoon Easy, Fresh Salsa (previous recipe) or a good organic salsa

1 teaspoon flaxseed oil

1. Cut the avocado in half, remove its pit, peel it, and, with a fork, mash it in a medium bowl.

2. Add the salsa and flaxseed oil, and mix together.

3. If you're using a food processor, combine the avocado and flaxseed oil in it. Use the pulse setting and blend until smooth. Add the salsa last, and pulse only once or twice to avoid liquefying it.

4. Pour the mixture into a serving dish and let the flavors mellow for 1 to 3 hours. Enjoy with Baked Corn Chips (page 118) or as a garnish for salads.

Makes 4 servings, each containing 42 calories, 1 gram of protein, 9 grams of carbohydrate, 0 grams of fat, and 2 grams of fiber

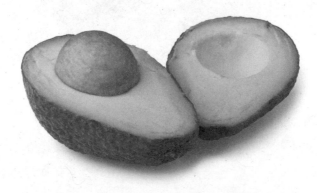

MANGO SALSA

A naturally sweet, juicy tropical fruit related to cashews and pistachios, mangoes contain ample vitamin C, beta-carotene, fiber, and minerals. Honey mangoes are a particularly sweet variety. The mango flesh has more fiber as you get down to the large, flat, and very slippery pit or seed. The beautiful golden-yellow color adds a bright accent to baked fish. Use this salsa to garnish fish or poultry, or as a dip for raw vegetables or Baked Corn Chips (page 118).

3 honey mangoes, peeled and chopped in 1/4-inch cubes

1 small to medium red onion, finely diced

1/2 cup cilantro, coarsely chopped

Pinch of cayenne pepper (optional)

1. Peel each mango one half at a time. Dice the mango flesh against the pit and then, by slicing parallel to it, carefully cut pieces of the fruit off of the pit.

2. In a medium bowl, add the onion and cilantro, and mix completely.

3. Add cayenne pepper to taste if desired. Start with a little and add more as needed, depending on your tolerance for hot spices and the intensity of your cayenne.

Makes almost 2 cups (4 servings), each serving containing 88 calories, 1 gram of protein, 23 grams of carbohydrate, 0 grams of fat, 3 grams of fiber, and 36 milligrams of vitamin C.

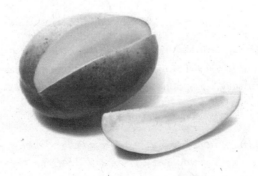

LIVER PÂTÉ

Give liver, a traditional health-building food, a try. The livers of healthy animals are a concentrated storehouse of all nutrients, in easily accessible forms. Organic, pasture-raised animals don't contain the toxins that feed-lot-raised animals encounter. Many people who don't like liver tell me they *love* this pâté. If you are sensitive to fermented soy, you can use salt instead of miso or try soy-free miso from South River Miso, made from chickpeas or aduki beans (see the resources for fermented foods). Serve warm or chilled on Flaxseed Crackers (page 112) (with spicy mustard) or crisp vegetable sticks.

4 tablespoons organic duck fat or palm oil

1 large organic onion, diced

1 pound organic chicken or duck liver

2 teaspoons thyme

2 teaspoons sage

2 teaspoons dulse granules (seaweed)

1/4 teaspoon fresh ground pepper (optional)

2 to 3 teaspoons brown (2-year-old) miso paste or 1/2 teaspoon unrefined salt

1. Melt half the duck fat or palm oil in a large skillet.

2. Using medium heat, sauté diced onion until translucent.

3. Add liver, reduce heat to low, and lightly sauté, approximately 5 to 10 minutes. As the liver cooks, add the thyme, sage, dulse, and, if desired, pepper. The liver is finished cooking when no red juice comes out of it.

4. Allow the liver-onion mixture to cool, and put it into a food processor.

5. Add the miso (or salt) and the rest of the duck fat or palm oil, and blend until smooth. If you need to avoid soy, substitute 1/2 teaspoon of salt for the miso and add 2 teaspoons more duck fat or palm oil.

6. Chill before serving or serve warm.

Makes about 16 servings, each 2-tablespoon serving containing 55 calories, 4 grams of protein, 4 grams of fat, and 1 gram of carbohydrate, plus 2,230 IU of vitamin A, 95 micrograms of folic acid, 2.7 micrograms of B12, 54 milligrams of potassium, and many trace minerals

SALADS AND DRESSINGS

Raw, fresh vegetable salads are cooling and refreshing. Raw vegetables contain many vitamins, some of which are destroyed by heat, and these sensitive vitamins are necessary for proper intestinal functioning. If you have constipation, be sure to include raw vegetables with every meal. If you have diarrhea, avoid raw foods for now, use the dressing on cooked foods, and then skip to the "Soups" section.

Though convenient, store-bought salad dressings contain many artificial or refined ingredients that can irritate the intestines. It's easy and fun to make your own dressings once every few weeks to use as needed.

If a recipe calls for lemon juice, don't use bottled or packaged lemon juice unless the label guarantees it's free of potentially irritating chemical preservatives. Fresh lemons are bursting with vitamin C complex and other antioxidants. Freshness is important; over time, the antioxidants in the juice are lost. If you are lucky enough have access to Meyer lemons, you'll marvel at their sweetness compared to commercially available lemons. If any of these dressing recipes is too sour for you, use less lemon or vinegar, and replace some of the volume with water.

MUSTARD DRESSING

1/4 to 1/2 cup lemon juice or organic apple cider vinegar

1/2 cup organic extra-virgin olive oil

1 to 3 teaspoons mustard powder or a teaspoon of organic prepared brown mustard

1. Combine all ingredients in a small bowl and whisk by hand, or mix in a blender on low speed. Transfer to a bottle and refrigerate.

2. Shake before using.

Makes 8 servings, each 2-tablespoon serving containing 83 calories, 0 grams of protein, 9 grams of fat, 1 gram of carbohydrate, and 0 grams of fiber

MISO DRESSING

This dressing is excellent on steamed vegetables or salads.

2 tablespoons brown miso paste (soy free, if needed; see resources)

1 teaspoon ginger powder or 2 teaspoons minced fresh ginger

4 tablespoons apple cider vinegar or lemon juice

2 tablespoons water

1/4 cup extra-virgin olive oil

4 tablespoons organic flaxseed oil

1. Using a blender, combine the miso, ginger, vinegar or lemon juice, and water.

2. Slowly add the olive oil while the blender is on low. The mixture should begin to thicken to a mayonnaise consistency.

3. Gently stir in the flaxseed oil.

4. Store the mixture immediately in the refrigerator.

Makes about 1 cup or 8 servings, each 2-tablespoon serving containing 129 calories, 14 grams of fat (including essential fatty acids), less than 1 gram of protein, and 1 gram of carbohydrate

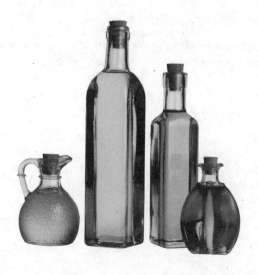

LEMON-GARLIC DRESSING

1/2 cup extra-virgin olive oil

1/3 cup lemon juice

1 to 2 cloves garlic, minced

1 teaspoon lemon zest

Pinch of salt

1. Combine all ingredients and blend until smooth.

2. Store the mixture in the refrigerator. Shake it before using.

Makes 6 servings, each 2-tablespoon serving containing 123 calories, 2 grams of fat, 1 gram of carbohydrate, 0 protein, and 0 fiber

SWEET CUCUMBER SALAD

Cucumbers are cooling and soothing, and because of their high water content, they can be very helpful for constipation. Armenian cucumbers are technically a type of melon and don't cause burping, as do some cucumber varieties. They have a thin, smooth, light-green skin. Cucumbers are in season from May to August. The cucumber peel contains most of the minerals and fiber, so choose unwaxed cucumbers for their nutrient-rich peels. Savor the crunchy, sweet, and sour flavor of this summer salad.

2 cucumbers, diced (Armenian preferred), about 2 cups

1 apple, diced

2 carrots, grated

2 lemons, juiced (about 2 ounces)

1. Combine the cucumbers, apple, and carrots in a medium bowl. Add the lemon juice and toss together.

2. Allow the mixture to marinate for 1 to 2 hours to let flavors mingle.

Makes approximately 3 cups or 6 servings, each serving containing 41 calories, 1 gram of protein, 10 grams of carbohydrate, 0 fat, and 2 grams of fiber

CONFETTI COLESLAW

This is a pretty summer slaw that's not only crunchy and colorful but also an excellent source of vitamin C and fiber. The acidic dressing turns the red cabbage a brilliant magenta, adding to this dish's festive quality. Try it with Savoy cabbage for its finer texture. Using stevia green-leaf powder will help balance the acidity of the lemon.

1/2 small red cabbage, shredded (1 1/2 cups)

1/2 small green cabbage, shredded (1 1/2 cups)

1 carrot, shredded

1 cup fresh cilantro or parsley, chopped

1 red bell pepper, diced (3/4 cup) (optional)

1/2 cup olive oil

1/4 cup lemon juice, or apple cider vinegar

1/8 teaspoon stevia green-leaf powder (optional)

1. Combine the shredded cabbages and carrot in a large bowl. Add the chopped cilantro or parsley, and bell pepper if desired.

2. Stir in the olive oil and lemon juice or vinegar.

3. Add stevia green-leaf powder a pinch at a time while stirring and tasting.

Makes 8 servings, each containing 155 calories, 2 grams of protein, 14 grams of fat, 8 grams of carbohydrate, 3 grams of fiber, and more than 100 percent of the recommended daily allowance (65 milligrams) of vitamin C

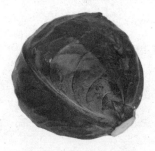

SAUERKRAUT

Sauerkraut is one of the oldest cultured foods. The canned version is nothing like the "live" version, which contains a wide variety of helpful bacteria, enzymes, and nutrients. Live, raw sauerkraut has been used for thousands of years to maintain health (Katz 2003). Add any grated vegetable for a variation, such as carrots, beets, onion, garlic, ginger, seaweed, or greens—or even apple. Caraway seed, dill, and fennel seed are classic additions. Daikon radish, carrot, and pepper are the basic ingredients of the Korean version of sauerkraut, known as *kimchi*.

2 heads cabbage (about 5 pounds)

3 tablespoons sea salt, Celtic salt, or Himalayan salt

1. Finely shred the cabbage and place it in a large bowl. Sprinkle in the salt as you go.

2. With your hands, a wooden pounder, or a potato masher, crush and mix the cabbage until some of the juices are released, resulting in a very wet mixture. The salty juice is the brine.

3. Place the cabbage and brine in a ceramic crock or large bowl. Place a large plate (to completely cover the cabbage) over the cabbage, and press it down until the brine covers the cabbage and plate. If there's not enough brine to cover the cabbage, add saltwater (1 tablespoon of salt dissolved in 1 pint of water).

4. Weight the plate down with a quart jar filled with water, and cover the crock and jar with a clean towel.

5. Leave the kraut to ferment in a cool, out-of-the-way part of your kitchen for up to four weeks, depending on the temperature. You can ferment sauerkraut for months in a cool environment, such as a basement or root cellar. Check the fermentation every few days. It should begin to get tangy and bubbly in about three to four days. Warmer temperatures speed up the fermentation process. If mold forms on top of the brine, scoop away as much as you can. It's not a problem as long as the cabbage stays below the liquid's surface. If the brine evaporates, add more saltwater. Remove the weight and the plate, and taste the kraut. The longer it ferments, the more sour and soft it becomes. You decide when it's to your liking. End the fermentation process by packing the kraut in jars and refrigerating it.

Makes about 8 cups, each 2-tablespoon serving containing 7 calories, 0 grams of protein, 2 grams of carbohydrate, 0 fat, and 1 gram of fiber

BEAN AND WHOLE-GRAIN SALAD

If you have any leftover cooked whole grain, this is a superquick meal. Using a food processor makes this salad even faster to prepare, and you can use it as a main dish for a summer lunch or dinner. When combined, legumes and whole grains provide all the essential amino acids to make complete protein.

1 cup organic brown rice (or quinoa, millet, buckwheat, or amaranth) or 2 cups cooked grain

2 1/2 cups water

1 cup cooked organic beans or lentils (or organic canned beans or frozen peas)

3 green onions, diced

1 stalk celery, diced

1 red pepper, diced

1 carrot, diced

2 tablespoons fresh parsley, cilantro, basil, or mint, chopped

1/2 cup sunflower seeds (or pumpkin or sesame seeds)

1/3 to 1/2 cup organic apple cider vinegar or fresh lemon juice

1/3 to 1/2 cup extra-virgin olive oil

Dulse granules or salt to taste

1. If you don't have any cooked leftover rice, combine the rice or grain of choice and water in a medium saucepan with a lid. Bring it to a boil, uncovered. Turn down the heat to a low simmer, and cover for 30 minutes, until the grain is tender and all the water is absorbed. Set aside to cool.

2. Chop the vegetables. You can use the pulse setting on your food processor.

3. If using canned beans, drain them.

4. Stir the rice, beans, or peas, and all remaining ingredients together in a large bowl. Add dulse or salt to taste.

5. Serve over lettuce leaves or steamed greens.

Makes 4 servings, each containing 636 calories, 20 grams of protein, 31 grams of fat, 75 grams of carbohydrate, and 10 grams of fiber

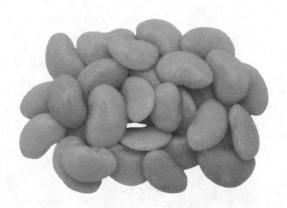

SPROUTED HUMMUS

Hummus is an ancient Mediterranean staple, usually made from cooked chick-peas and sesame tahini, though many variations exist. This raw hummus is bursting with enzymes, protein, minerals, vitamins, and fiber, and can be used as a dip, dressing, or entree. Serve it with carrot sticks, celery sticks, cucumber slices, or other raw vegetables.

1 1/2 cups bean sprouts (page 108)

1/2 cup sunflower seed sprouts or tahini

2 cloves garlic

1/4 cup lemon juice

1/4 cup olive oil

Salt to taste

Dulse granules (seaweed) for garnish

1. Place all ingredients except salt and dulse in a blender and purée until smooth. If it's too thick, add some water to help blend.

2. Add salt to taste and serve in a bowl with a sprinkle of dulse for color.

Makes 6 servings, each containing 334 calories, 12 grams of protein, 18 grams of fat, 34 grams of carbohydrate, and 10 grams of fiber

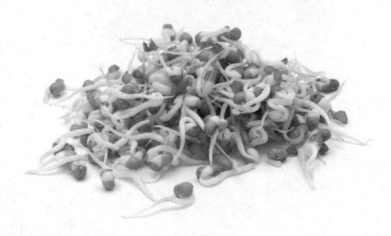

SARDINE SALAD

This is a tasty way to get leafy greens and omega-3-rich fish in one fast meal. The greens, fish, and dressing can travel separately so you can easily assemble this salad just before eating. Sardines are small fish that are full of protein, calcium, and essential omega-3 fatty acids. We need omega-3 fatty acids to reduce inflammation. Until the last 50 years, sardines and other small fish were a regular part of the diet. They are plentiful and don't accumulate mercury due to their small size.

2 to 3 cups organic salad-green mix or lettuce

1/4 to 1/2 cup sliced carrots, snow peas, sprouts, celery, cucumber, or other fresh vegetable (optional)

1 (3.75 ounce) can sardines, packed in water (with the bones, a great calcium source)

2 tablespoons dressing, such as Mustard Dressing (page 123), Miso Dressing (page 124), or Lemon-Garlic Dressing (page 125).

1. Wash salad greens, and spin or pat dry. Place the greens and any other fresh, crunchy vegetables you like in a bowl.

2. Open and drain the canned fish, and add it to the greens.

3. Top with the dressing of your choice. Relax and enjoy.

Makes 1 serving containing 332 calories, 26 grams of protein, 20 grams of fat, 14 grams of carbohydrate, 5 grams of fiber, and 435 milligrams of omega-3 fatty acids

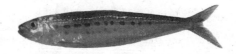

VEGETABLE DISHES

Make vegetables three-quarters of each meal for the optimal amount of vitamins, minerals, and fiber. These are easy recipes the whole family will enjoy.

BAKED WINTER SQUASH

Squash is a great source of potassium, vitamin B2, folic acid, beta-carotene, vitamins C and K, and trace minerals, including copper and manganese. Winter squashes have thick, inedible skin and tough seeds, and will keep in a cool, dry place for up to six months. Choose any variety of organic winter squash, such as acorn, butternut, buttercup, carnival, delicata, turban, spaghetti, or *kabocha* (Japanese pumpkin). Look for squashes with smooth, unblemished skin. Some have a yellowish spot, which can indicate ripeness. For a festive side dish, cut the baked squash in half, scoop out the seeds, and stuff it with rice or Millet-Amaranth Pilaf (page 138).

1 winter squash, whole (1 to 5 pounds, depending on variety)

Garnishes: cinnamon, cardamom, or pumpkin pie spice; coconut butter or Fabulous Flaxseed and Pumpkin Seed Spread (page 115); or Rose-Hip Spread (page 114)

1. Preheat oven to 350°F. Wash the exterior of the squash. Pierce the skin with a sharp knife (to prevent it from bursting open unexpectedly during cooking). Place the whole squash on a baking dish and bake it until you can insert a fork, approximately 1 hour. Very large squashes may take even longer. Remove the squash from the oven and allow it to cool enough to be handled.

2. Cut the squash in half and gently scoop out the seeds. (You can eat these like pumpkin seeds, whole or hulled.)

3. Serve the squash hot, sprinkled with spice and garnished with coconut cream concentrate, rose-hip spread, or both.

Total yield depends on size of squash, each 1-cup serving containing 76 calories, 2 grams of protein, 1 gram of fat, 18 grams of carbohydrate, and 6 grams of fiber

ROASTED ROOT VEGETABLES

Roasting intensifies the sweet flavor of vegetables. Roasting time varies depending on the size of the vegetable pieces, the hardness of the vegetable, and the temperature of the oven. Try red beets or Spanish black radishes. Both are excellent for the liver and digestion.

3 to 8 beets, carrots, Spanish black radishes, daikon radishes, turnips, or any combination thereof (about 1 pound)

1 tablespoon olive oil

1 teaspoon thyme or oregano

1/2 teaspoon rosemary

1. Preheat oven to 300°F.

2. Chop the root vegetables into 1-inch chunks. Put them in a baking dish, and toss with the olive oil and spices until they are coated with both.

3. Bake uncovered in the oven for 30 to 45 minutes.

4. Remove from oven and turn the pieces over, checking for tenderness. When a fork goes in easily, they are done.

5. Serve hot or cold.

Total yield is variable, with 2 roasted beets containing 44 calories, 2 grams of protein, 0 fat, 10 grams of carbohydrate, and 2 grams of fiber

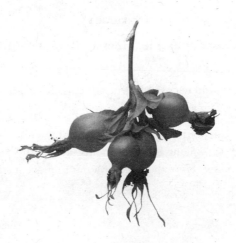

LAURA'S FANTASTIC GREENS

Even those who have never liked green leafy vegetables love this recipe. Greens are a rich source of vitamins and trace minerals, especially beta-carotene, calcium, and potassium, which are necessary for proper bowel function.

Kale is especially good for the liver. Its carotenes and bioflavonoids help the lungs, eyes, immune system, and digestive system, and it protects against colon cancer. It contains considerable calcium, magnesium, and iron. All green vegetables contain chlorophyll, but the darker green varieties of kale and collards contain even more. Kale has a warming thermal nature and a sweet-bitter-pungent flavor. Shiitake mushrooms are beneficial to the stomach and are said to be a natural source of *interferon*, a protein involved in the immune response. Mushrooms are a good source of the mineral *germanium*, also needed for good immune functioning. Use any variety of kale, collards, mustard greens, bok choy, or cabbage. Keep in mind that these sturdier greens lose only about one-third of their original volume when cooked. If you decide to use chard, spinach, or dandelion instead, start with three or four times as much, because they cook down to only a third to a quarter of their original volume.

> **1 bunch kale or other sturdy greens (about 10 to 12 ounces)**
>
> **1 to 2 tablespoons extra-virgin olive, coconut, or palm oil, or chicken fat**
>
> **1 small onion, diced**
>
> **1/2 cup mushrooms, sliced (shiitake mushrooms are especially good)**
>
> **1/2 cup stock, bone broth, or water**
>
> **1 tablespoon wheat-free soy sauce**
>
> **Lemon juice or apple cider vinegar, flaxseed oil, or both to garnish**

1. Wash the greens and remove the central stems. Break greens into bite-sized pieces with your fingers.

2. Heat a large skillet or pot to medium, and add the oil or fat to lightly coat the pan. Sauté the onions and mushrooms until both just begin to brown. Add 1 to 2 tablespoons of the stock or water to prevent sticking.

3. Add the greens and stir quickly so that all become bright green.

4. Mix the stock or water with soy sauce, add it to the greens, and cover it. Let it simmer until the greens achieve the desired tenderness and most, but not all, of the liquid is gone. (Spinach and chard cook in about 5 minutes; kale and collards take up to 20 minutes.)

5. Serve immediately. If desired, dress each serving with lemon juice or vinegar, flaxseed oil, or both.

Makes 3 to 4 one-cup servings, depending on type of greens, each serving containing 96 calories, 4 grams of protein, 3 grams of fat, 15 grams of carbohydrate, and 4 grams of fiber

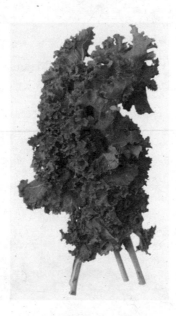

MASHED GARLIC CAULIFLOWER

This flavorful dish is a unique replacement for mashed potatoes if you are sensitive to nightshade vegetables (such as potato, tomato, eggplant, and pepper), or just want a low-carbohydrate option. Cauliflower and garlic are both excellent for liver detoxification. When you need comfort food, serve this dish with Turkey Meat Loaf (page 156) and use the meat drippings as gravy.

1 large cauliflower (about 1 pound)

5 cloves garlic (peeled)

1 1/2 tablespoons duck fat or chicken fat

Pinch of salt

1. Cut the cauliflower into florets.

2. Steam the cauliflower and garlic cloves for 10 minutes, until the cauliflower stems are tender when pierced by a fork.

3. Put cauliflower, garlic, and fat in a food processor or blender, and whip until smooth. Add salt to taste. Serve as you would mashed potatoes.

Makes 6 servings, each containing 56 calories, 2 grams of protein, 3 grams of fat, 6 grams of carbohydrate, and 2 grams of fiber

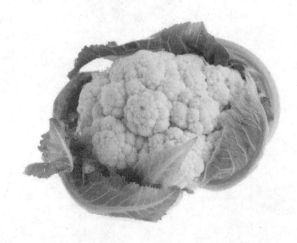

COLLARD NOODLES

This is a simple and nutritious substitution for linguini noodles. When I had to give up pasta, I thought I had to give up twirling, but these "noodles" twirl just like the real thing. This is a wonderful side dish for Chicken Italiano (page 157). Enjoy.

1 bunch collard greens, about 8 large leaves

Lemon juice and flaxseed oil as garnish

1. Remove the central stem from each collard leaf, cutting each leaf in half lengthwise. They should be long, flat half-ovals. Stack all the greens and roll them into a fat cylinder.

2. Using a sharp knife, cut the roll crosswise into thin strips, each about 1/4-inch wide. This should create long, thin strips of collard greens.

3. Unroll these strips into a steamer and steam for 15 to 25 minutes, depending on the thickness of the collards.

4. Serve as you would noodles, with any sauce or dressing, or with just a garnish of lemon juice and flaxseed oil.

Makes 4 servings, each containing 49 calories, 4 grams of protein, 1 gram of fat, 9 grams of carbohydrate, and 5 grams of fiber

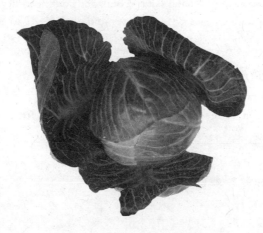

GLUTEN-FREE GRAIN SIDE DISHES

If you are sensitive to gluten-containing grains, such as wheat, rye, barley, Kamut, spelt, and oats, use these gluten-free whole grains: amaranth, buckwheat, corn, millet, quinoa, rice, and teff. Oats are usually contaminated with wheat, so if you want to use oats, be sure to get certified gluten-free (such as Bob's Red Mill). Here are some healthy ways to serve whole grains.

MILLET-AMARANTH PILAF

Use this colorful dish to stuff a Baked Winter Squash (page 132), or serve it as a side dish. *Variation:* Use the tiny Ethiopian seed, teff, instead of amaranth.

3 cups Mineral-Rich Bone Broth (page 141) or water

Pinch of sea salt

1/2 cup organic millet

1/2 cup organic amaranth

1 1/2 cups organic peas, fresh or frozen

1/4 to 1/2 cup raw pumpkin seeds or sliced almonds

1 red sweet bell pepper, finely diced

1. Bring the broth or water and salt to a boil, and add the millet and amaranth. Turn the heat down to a simmer. Cover and cook for 10 to 15 minutes.

2. Add the peas. Cover again and simmer for 10 more minutes, until the water is completely absorbed and the grains are tender.

3. Stir in the pumpkin seeds or sliced almonds and the red bell pepper, and remove the mixture from the heat. Let it sit, covered, for an additional 5 to 10 minutes.

Makes 8 servings, each containing 227 calories, 9 grams of protein, 6 grams of fat, 37 grams of carbohydrate, and 5 grams of fiber

KASHA

This is an old Russian favorite you can eat anytime as a side dish to any meal, or with Beet Soup (page 146). Gluten free, buckwheat is not a grain but a seed, and is related to rhubarb and sorrel. It has a rich, nutty flavor.

1 1/2 cups raw buckwheat groats

1 egg, beaten lightly

3 cups Mineral-Rich Bone Broth (page 141), or water

Pinch of salt and pepper

1. Heat a large cast-iron skillet over medium-high heat, and add the buckwheat. Gently toast the groats for about 3 minutes, until they just begin to brown slightly.

2. Add the egg and stir it in thoroughly until it's totally dry.

3. Add the broth or water. Cover the mixture and simmer it on low for 15 to 20 minutes, until the liquid is absorbed and the buckwheat is tender. Add salt and pepper to taste.

Makes 6 to 8 servings, each 1/2-cup serving containing 162 calories, 7 grams of protein, 2 grams of fat, 31 grams of carbohydrate, and 4 grams of fiber

POLENTA

This way to make polenta (Italian cornmeal mush) is fast and guarantees no lumps. Serve with pesto, tomato sauce, or Easy, Fresh Salsa (page 119).

1 cup coarse cornmeal

3 cups Mineral-Rich Bone Broth (page 141), or water

1 tablespoon *gomasio* (sesame salt)

1 tablespoon organic extra-virgin olive oil

1. Mix cornmeal and cold broth or water in a medium saucepan. Stir the mixture over medium heat until it thickens.

2. Stir in the gomasio and the olive oil, cover the mixture, and set aside for 10 minutes.

Serves 6, each half-cup serving containing 101 calories, 2 grams of protein, 4 grams of fat, 16 grams of carbohydrate, and 2 grams of fiber

SIMPLE FRIED RICE

Though not authentically Chinese, this dish is tasty and satisfying. It is a very good source of vitamin A and manganese.

1 tablespoon palm or coconut oil

1 egg

1 (10-ounce) package frozen organic peas and carrots

1/4 cup Mineral-Rich Bone Broth (recipe follows) or water

2 cups cooked long-grain brown rice

1 to 2 tablespoons organic, wheat-free tamari (soy sauce)

1. In a frying pan over medium heat, scramble the egg in the oil.

2. Add the peas and carrots, and the broth or water. Let this mixture simmer for 3 to 5 minutes, until the vegetables are no longer frozen.

3. Quickly stir in the cooked rice and soy sauce.

4. Serve hot.

Serves 4, each half-cup serving containing 198 calories, 7 grams of protein, 6 grams of fat, 31 grams of carbohydrate, and 4 grams of fiber

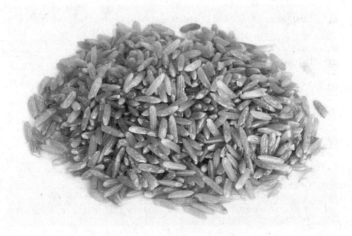

SOUPS

Soups are a traditional way to nourish body and soul. Nutrients in a solution are more digestible and absorbable. Soups are truly healing and very easy to assemble. You can also make them in big batches, freeze single servings, and quickly heat them on the stove when you need them.

MINERAL-RICH BONE BROTH

Use this broth to cook soups or grains, or drink it warm anytime to improve absorbable mineral intake. Traditional people used bone broth to cure almost everything. As a low-calorie source of minerals and protein, broth is hard to beat. I save the bones from my roasts and freeze them, along with eggshells, until I have about half a stockpot full. Any fat on the bones improves the flavor. Once you've chilled the broth, you can skim off the fat and save it to sauté eggs or vegetables.

3 to 5 pounds bones, such as turkey, beef, lamb, or chicken (organic or pasture raised)

6 to 12 eggshells, cleaned (optional)

Water to cover bones

2 to 3 tablespoons vinegar or lemon juice

1 to 4 tablespoons dulse (seaweed)

Vegetable parings (optional)

1. Place the bones and shells in a stockpot. Cover them completely with water.

2. Add the vinegar or lemon juice.

3. Bring the mixture to a boil and skim off any froth that comes to the top. Add the dulse. Cover and simmer very slowly for 12 to 36 hours.

4. Add vegetable parings, if desired, and simmer for another hour.

5. Strain the stock into quart or pint containers. Store frozen for up to three months.

Makes variable yield, each 1/2 cup serving containing 23 calories, 3 grams of protein, 1 gram of fat, 0 carbohydrate, and 0 fiber

VEGETABLE STOCK

You can freeze this tasty stock in 1-cup freezer jars or ice cube trays. Cone-shaped freezer jars allow you to easily remove the stock while it's still frozen.

All fresh organic vegetables are especially good sources of potassium, calcium, and magnesium, so this stock is rich in minerals, but it contains little protein. Use it to replace water in recipes; it will add flavor along with the minerals. You can also use it to sauté vegetables or cook grains.

This broth keeps for up to three days in the refrigerator or three months in the freezer.

1 bunch parsley

1 onion, chopped

2 to 3 stems celery, both stalks and leaves, chopped

1 pound green beans (about 2 1/2 cups)

2 carrots, chopped

1/2 teaspoon thyme

1 teaspoon basil

1 teaspoon rosemary

3 to 6 cloves garlic

2 bay leaves

1 teaspoon dulse granules

1/2 teaspoon sea salt

Water, enough to totally cover the vegetables, about 4 to 7 cups

1. Put all ingredients together in a soup pot and bring to a boil.

2. Reduce heat to a low simmer for 45 minutes to 1 hour. Remove it from the heat and allow it to cool.

3. Strain the mixture into a large jar or several smaller ones. Leave the containers about 10 percent empty to allow the liquid to expand as it freezes. Close them and allow them to cool before refrigerating or freezing.

Variable yield, each 1-cup serving containing 12 calories, 0 protein, 0 fat, 3 grams of carbohydrate, and 0 fiber

CHICKEN-VEGETABLE SOUP

An old-fashioned favorite made easy, this soup is a standard for anyone with digestive or immunity problems. Soothing and comforting, it's a good way to get the vitamin A precursor beta-carotene. The vegetables are cooked till soft for easier digestion. The minerals in the vegetables and proteins in the chicken partly dissolve, making them more available for absorption. If you have trouble chewing or swallowing, blend the soup. Use any vegetables on hand.

1 pound organic chicken legs (about 2 legs)

4 carrots, cut in chunks

1 large onion, chopped

3 stalks celery, chopped

4 cloves garlic, chopped or whole

2 cups green beans

2 quarts Mineral-Rich Bone Broth (page 141) or Vegetable Stock (previous recipe)

1 teaspoon dulse granules

Pinch of salt

1 bunch parsley, chopped fine

1. Place all ingredients in a large soup pot, except the parsley, and bring to a boil.

2. Cover and simmer for 45 minutes, until the chicken is thoroughly cooked and falling apart. Add the chopped parsley and simmer for 5 minutes.

Serves 6, each serving containing 201 calories, 23 grams of protein, 8 grams of fat, 11 grams of carbohydrate, and 3 grams of fiber, plus 6,574 IU of beta-carotene

JAPANESE-STYLE FISH SOUP

This satisfying soup provides excellent nutrition for a light dinner. Fresh halibut is especially good in this recipe.

1 piece of gingerroot, 1 inch long, minced

1 small onion, diced

3 cloves garlic, sliced

3 cups Mineral-Rich Bone Broth (page 141) or Vegetable Stock (page 142)

1/2 pound fish, cut into 1-inch chunks

2 carrots, chopped

1 cup cabbage or other green leafy vegetable, chopped

1 cup broccoli florets

1/4 cup nori seaweed, shredded (about 1 to 2 sheets)

2 teaspoons miso

1 green onion, chopped

1. In a medium saucepan, add the ginger, onion, garlic, and broth. Bring this mixture to a boil and simmer for 10 minutes.

2. Add the fish and the rest of the vegetables (except the green onion), and simmer for another 10 minutes or until the fish is done.

3. Remove the soup from the heat. Place some of the broth in serving bowls and stir 1 teaspoon of the miso into each bowl.

4. Garnish with chopped green onion and serve.

Makes 2 servings, each serving containing 257 calories, 33 grams of protein, 3 grams of fat, 27 grams of carbohydrate, 8 grams of fiber, and 1,027 milligrams of potassium.

THAI CHICKEN SOUP

Make this soup as spicy or as bland as you want by adjusting the amount of curry paste. Use coconut cream concentrate instead of canned coconut milk, which contains guar gum and preservatives that can irritate the intestines.

4 boneless chicken thighs (about 1 pound)

1 quart Mineral-Rich Bone Broth (page 141)

1 piece of lemongrass, 6 inches long

1 piece of gingerroot, 1/2-inch long, minced

2 zucchini, chopped

2 tablespoons coconut cream concentrate or coconut butter

2 tablespoons warm water

1 to 3 teaspoons green Thai curry paste or 1 to 3 chiles

1 bunch fresh cilantro, chopped

1. Brown and then sauté the chicken thighs until cooked thoroughly. Cut the chicken into 11/2-inch chunks.

2. Place the broth, lemongrass, ginger, and zucchini in a saucepan and heat for 10 minutes.

3. Mix the coconut cream concentrate with the warm water to make coconut milk.

4. Mix the curry paste with the coconut milk by mixing a small bit of the milk with the paste and then adding the rest of the coconut milk. If using peppers instead of paste, chop them and add to the coconut milk.

5. Remove the lemongrass from the broth with tongs or a fork, and add the coconut milk and the curry paste or peppers to the soup.

6. Garnish with fresh cilantro and serve.

Makes 4 servings, each containing 334 calories, 20 grams of protein, 26 grams of fat, 9 grams of carbohydrate, and 1 gram of fiber

BEET SOUP

A good source of minerals and phytonutrients, beets help improve the function of the liver and bowel. Serve with Kasha (page 139).

> **2 beets (about 6 ounces), with or without the greens**
>
> **2 carrots, chopped**
>
> **1 onion, diced**
>
> **1 bunch kale (if no beet greens)**
>
> **2 cloves garlic, minced**
>
> **1 piece of fresh ginger, 1/2-inch long, minced**
>
> **3 cups Mineral-Rich Bone Broth (page 141), Vegetable Stock (page 142), or water**
>
> **2 teaspoons dill leaf, dried**
>
> **1/2 teaspoon dulse granules**
>
> **1/4 teaspoon sea salt, if using water instead of broth or stock**
>
> **2 tablespoons apple cider vinegar**

1. Scrub the beets, slice into 1/4-inch-thick slices, and put them in a large saucepan or soup pot.

2. Add the rest of the vegetables to the beets. Add broth or stock, dill, dulse, and vinegar, and simmer for 45 minutes or until the beets are tender. Salt to taste.

3. Serve hot or cold.

Makes 2 beautiful servings, each containing 154 calories, 8 grams of protein, 2 grams of fat, 32 grams of carbohydrate, and 9 grams of fiber

WINTER SQUASH SOUP

The orange color of this creamy, smooth soup is perfect on a cool fall evening. Try it with butternut, acorn, turban, sugar pie, or Japanese pumpkin (kabocha) squash.

1 winter squash (about 3 to 5 pounds), baked and peeled

4 carrots, chopped

1 onion, diced

1 to 2 tablespoons coconut or palm oil

1/2 teaspoon cumin powder

1/4 teaspoon ginger powder

1/4 teaspoon turmeric powder

1/4 teaspoon coriander, ground

1/4 teaspoon cardamom, ground

1 cup Mineral-Rich Bone Broth (page 141), Vegetable Stock (page 142), or water

Pinch of salt and pepper (optional)

Pumpkin seeds or flaxseeds for garnish (optional)

1. Bake the squash whole as described in the Baked Winter Squash recipe (page 132). Let it cool, and remove the skin and seeds.

2. Sauté the carrots and onion in the coconut or palm oil for 15 minutes, until tender.

3. In a food processor, combine the cooked squash, carrots and onion, spices, and stock. Blend until smooth. Add salt and pepper to taste, and increase the quantities of any or all of the spices as your taste dictates.

4. Return the soup to the saucepan and heat.

5. Garnish with ground pumpkin seeds (or flaxseeds) and serve hot.

Serves 4, each serving containing 141 calories, 3 grams of protein, 4 grams of fat, 26 grams of carbohydrate, and 8 grams of fiber, plus vitamins C, B6, and K, and potassium (1,137 milligrams)

ENTREES

Eat these main dishes at any time of day. Cook enough to make leftovers for the next two meals to save time in the kitchen. Cook once; eat thrice. Though most of these recipes are designed to reduce time spent preparing food, they are still nutrient dense. Use them in your rotation diet as is or with minor substitutions, depending on your needs.

FAST BEANS AND CORN

This dish has a prep time of 10 minutes or less. It's good on salad greens, or eat it as a party dip with raw vegetables or Baked Corn Chips (page 118).

1 (12-ounce) can organic black beans (or any bean except soybeans)

1 (10-ounce) package frozen organic corn kernels

1 (12-ounce) jar organic salsa (your preferred level of spiciness)

1. Combine all ingredients in a saucepan. Stir together over medium heat until the corn is no longer frozen.

2. Serve hot or cold.

Makes 4 to 6 servings, each generous serving containing 170 calories, 9 grams of protein, 1 gram of fat, 34 grams of carbohydrate, and 8 grams of fiber

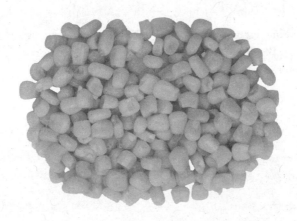

SPAGHETTI-SQUASH FRITTATA

Frittatas are the perfect thing for a quick, spur-of-the-moment breakfast, lunch, or supper. They're even good cold, so you can pack them for a picnic or a brown-bag lunch. Substitute zucchini or other summer vegetables for the spaghetti squash if you desire.

1 spaghetti squash (about 3 to 4 pounds), baked

4 eggs, beaten lightly

4 tablespoons fresh parsley, chopped

3 tablespoons gomasio (sesame salt)

1/2 teaspoon pepper (optional)

1/8 teaspoon cayenne (optional)

1/2 teaspoon dulse granules

1 cup red onion, finely chopped

3 to 4 garlic cloves, minced

1 to 2 tablespoons olive oil

1. Preheat oven to 350°F.

2. Bake spaghetti squash whole as described in the Baked Winter Squash recipe (page 132), and allow it to cool.

3. Cut squash in half, and use a fork to remove and separate the noodle-like strands. (You'll have about 3 to 4 cups of squash.)

4. Combine squash, eggs, parsley, gomasio, pepper, cayenne, and dulse in a large mixing bowl.

5. In a large, deep cast-iron skillet or saucepan, sauté the onion and garlic in the olive oil. Add in the squash-egg mixture and cook, covered, over low heat for about 10 minutes.

6. Transfer the iron skillet to the oven for 15 to 20 minutes, until the top of the vegetable mixture is browned and the liquid has cooked off. It's done when an inserted fork comes out clean.

Makes 4 servings, each containing 213 calories, 9 grams of protein, 15 grams of fat, 12 grams of carbohydrate, and 3 grams of fiber

SHRIMP CURRY

A blend of several Indian spices, curry powder comes in many varieties and levels of spiciness. I like the mild madras type I get in bulk at a local health-food store. Since I buy it in bulk, I can smell how fresh (and spicy) it is before purchasing it. Sun-dried tomatoes add a more intense flavor than fresh tomato; use either. Cooking the shrimp gently at a low temperature makes them tender and juicy.

1 pound frozen shrimp, thawed, shelled and deveined

1/2 cup sun-dried tomatoes, soaked in 1/2 cup water, or 1/2 cup fresh tomato, diced

1 to 2 tablespoons coconut oil for sautéing

1 onion, diced

2 celery stalks, diced

2 carrots, sliced

4 teaspoons curry powder

1 teaspoon dulse granules

1 cup frozen peas (about 5 ounces)

1 to 2 tablespoons coconut cream concentrate, dissolved in 3/4 cup warm water, or 1/2 cup coconut milk

1 bunch (about 3/4 cup) basil, mint, or cilantro leaves, or any combination thereof, chopped (optional)

1. Rinse the shrimp in a colander and set aside.

2. After soaking the sun-dried tomatoes in water, reserve the soak water to use later.

3. In a large, deep skillet or saucepan, sauté the onion, celery, and carrots in the coconut oil over medium heat until tender, about 10 minutes.

4. Stir in the curry powder and dulse. Add the soaked tomatoes and their soak water. (If using fresh tomato, add it at the end, when you add the basil.) Add the peas and drained shrimp, and cover.

5. Melt the coconut cream concentrate in warm water and add it.

6. Turn down the heat to low and simmer until the peas have become bright green and are no longer frozen, and the shrimp is opaque and not translucent.

7. Add the chopped basil, mint, or cilantro, or all of these, and add fresh tomatoes, if desired.

8. Remove from the heat and cover for 5 minutes.

9. Serve over Collard Noodles (page 137), brown rice, or steamed greens.

Makes 4 servings, each containing 258 calories, 27 grams of protein, 9 grams of fat, 19 grams of carbohydrate, and 5 grams of fiber

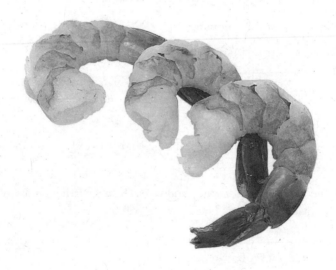

SHRIMP STIR-FRY

A stir-fry is a tasty way to eat more vegetables. Use whatever vegetables are on hand. Cabbage, carrots, onions, garlic, and ginger are staples you can depend on. Substitute for the shrimp any poultry or meat you prefer.

2 to 3 tablespoons coconut or palm oil, or chicken fat

1/2 pound shrimp, fresh or frozen, rinsed and drained

4 cloves garlic, chopped

1 piece of gingerroot, 1/2-inch long, minced

1 onion, diced

2 stalks celery, chopped

2 carrots, sliced

1 1/2 cups broccoli or cauliflower, cut in small florets

1 small cabbage, shredded

1 cup broth, stock, or water

Wheat-free tamari (soy sauce)

1. In a large, deep skillet or wok, at medium-high temperature, heat the oil or fat. Add the shrimp, garlic, ginger, onion, and celery, and sauté until the onion is translucent.

2. Add the carrots, broccoli, and cabbage, and stir briskly until the cabbage and broccoli turn bright green.

3. Add the broth, stock, or water, and cover. Sauté, stirring occasionally, for approximately 10 to 15 minutes, until the cabbage is done to taste.

4. Serve hot. Garnish with wheat-free soy sauce and serve over Collard Noodles (page 137), brown rice, or spaghetti squash.

Serves 4, each serving containing 213 calories, 15 grams of protein, 8 grams of fat, 22 grams of carbohydrate, and 6 grams of fiber

BAKED FISH

Most people overcook fish. Cooking at temperatures above 300°F releases the fishy odor, overcooking the fish and drying it out. The following gentle method keeps the fish moist and enhances its delicate flavor. I prefer using a glass baking pan, because it insulates rather than conducts heat. Wrapping the fish in nori sheets helps preserve moistness, just as wrapping fish in parchment does, and also adds important minerals. Bake fish in a coating of dulse, nori, or kelp granules, dill leaf, garlic powder, ginger, paprika, or a combination of these, depending on your preference. Be creative.

1 pound ocean fish fillets, such as halibut, black cod, pacific salmon, tuna, or snapper

2 teaspoons ginger powder or other spice

Dulse granules or sheets of sushi nori (to completely cover fillets)

Fresh lemon, cut in wedges

1. Preheat oven to 300°F.

2. Rinse the fish fillets under cold water. Place fish in the baking pan. Sprinkle with your preferred spices. Wrap each fillet in a nori sheet, or cover thickly with dulse granules.

3. Bake at 300°F for 15 minutes for each 1/2-inch thickness of the fillet.

4. Garnish with lemon wedges.

Serving size, 3 ounces, with different nutrient levels for each kind of fish, though all are high in protein, averaging about 7 grams per ounce, with almost no fat or carbohydrates

SLOW-COOKED TURKEY THIGH

The beauty of this recipe is that you can let it cook while you are away, asleep, or just busy doing something else. If you have a slow cooker or an oven with an automatic timer, you can come home after a hard day's work to a house filled with the aroma of a hot and ready dinner. After absorbing some of the meat juices and spices, this dish should be very tender and savory.

Each oven, slow cooker, and casserole dish is different, so the first time you try this recipe, it's best if you monitor the process to make sure the dish doesn't dry out or burn. If you're using an oven, I recommend using a covered glass casserole dish, because it distributes the heat and cooks more slowly and evenly. Metal roasting pans conduct heat, making the roast tend to burn unless you add plenty of liquid. Include stock or water if using a metal roasting pan or if you intend to use longer cooking times.

Try this dish with other root vegetables, such as beets, turnips, black radishes, or daikon radishes. Steam some asparagus or broccoli, toss a salad, and you have a healthy, colorful meal.

3 large carrots, cut into large chunks

1 to 3 free-range or organic turkey thighs (2 to 4 pounds)

Pinch of dulse granules (seaweed)

2 teaspoons garlic powder or 6 whole cloves, peeled

1 tablespoon dried sage, thyme, oregano, or parsley

1 large onion, cut into 1/4-inch-thick slices

Mineral-Rich Bone Broth (page 141), Vegetable Stock (page 142), or water, if needed for longer roasting

1. Put the carrots in a covered glass casserole or slow cooker. Place the turkey, skin-side up, on top of the carrots. Sprinkle the dulse and other spices on the turkey. Arrange the onion slices to cover the turkey.

2. If cooking this dish for more than 8 hours, add enough broth or water to cover the bottom of the pan to about 1/2-inch deep. Most, but not all, of the liquid will cook down. If cooking for 3 to 5 hours, set the oven to 250 to 275°F. If cooking for longer than 5 hours, set the oven to 200 to 225°F.

3. Cover the dish securely and put it in the oven, or use the slow cooker on medium or low.

4. The roast is done when a meat thermometer shows 190°F or the meat is so tender and juicy, it falls apart.

Makes 4 to 8 servings, each containing 231 calories, 20 grams of protein, 14 grams of fat, 6 grams of carbohydrate, and 2 grams of fiber

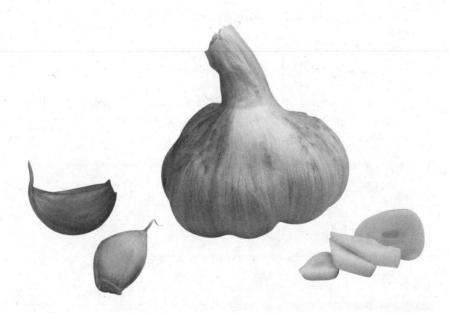

TURKEY MEAT LOAF

Deeply satisfying and flavorful, this dish is great served with Mashed Garlic Cauliflower (page 136). Use the broth that forms after the loaf is baked as gravy on the mashed-potato-like cauliflower. The mushrooms add moistness and enhance the flavor wonderfully. Adjust the garlic to your taste. One whole head of garlic sounds like a lot, but it's hardly noticeable once cooked. Using a food processor speeds the preparation considerably.

15 crimini mushrooms (3 ounces)

1/4 to 3/4 head garlic (4 to 10 cloves or about 1 ounce), peeled

1/3 cup olive oil

1 teaspoon thyme, dried

1 teaspoon salt

4 carrots (3 1/2 cups), shredded

2 pounds ground turkey-thigh meat

Pinch dulse or paprika

1. Preheat oven to 350°F.

2. In a food processor or blender, combine the mushrooms, garlic, olive oil, thyme, and salt, and blend to a paste. Add the carrots and continue blending.

3. In a large bowl, thoroughly mix the ground turkey with the carrot-mushroom-garlic paste.

4. Put the mixture into a covered glass casserole dish and form it into a loaf. Sprinkle with dulse or paprika if desired.

5. Cover and bake at 350°F for 1 hour, until a meat thermometer reads 190°F.

Makes 8 generous servings, each containing 279 calories, 21 grams of protein, 18 grams of fat, 7 grams of carbohydrate, and 2 grams of fiber

CHICKEN ITALIANO

This is so easy to make, yet tastes as if you worked all day.

2 chicken legs or 4 chicken thighs (about 1 pound)

6 cloves garlic, peeled

1 small onion, diced

1/4 pound crimini (brown) mushrooms, sliced (optional)

1 small (6-ounce) jar organic tomato paste

1 (29-ounce) can organic tomato purée

2 teaspoons oregano, dried

2 teaspoons thyme, dried

1 teaspoon dulse granules

1. Preheat oven to 275°F.

2. Put chicken legs in a 2-quart glass casserole dish with a lid. Add garlic, onion, and mushrooms if desired.

3. In a medium bowl, whisk together the tomato paste and purée with the oregano, thyme, and dulse. Pour the tomato mixture over the chicken, covering it completely.

4. Cover and bake for 3 hours, until the meat separates from the bone or a meat thermometer reads 190°F.

5. Serve over baked spaghetti squash or Collard Noodles (page 137).

Makes 4 servings, each containing 288 calories, 22 grams of protein, 10 grams of fat, 31 grams of carbohydrate, and 7 grams of fiber

LAMB-FENNEL STEW

Inexpensive cuts of lamb are more flavorful than expensive cuts, and become very tender in this slow-roasted recipe. Fennel improves the digestion. If you can't find shallots, substitute a medium onion.

> **1 large fennel bulb, sliced**
>
> **3 pounds lamb shanks or shoulder-blade chops (with bones)**
>
> **3 medium shallots, sliced**
>
> **1 (10-ounce) package frozen organic peas**
>
> **1 pint Mineral-Rich Bone Broth (page 141), Vegetable Stock (page 142), or water**
>
> **1/2 teaspoon salt**

1. Preheat oven to 250°F.

2. Line the bottom of a 2-quart covered glass casserole or slow cooker with the fennel slices. Add the lamb, shallots (or onion), peas, broth, and salt.

3. Cover and bake for 3 hours, until the meat is so tender that it separates from the bones or a meat thermometer reads 150°F.

Makes 4 servings, each containing 301 calories, 27 grams of protein, 15 grams of fat, 16 grams of carbohydrate, and 5 grams of fiber

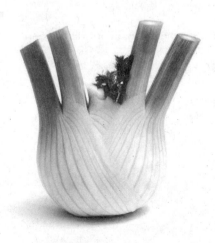

LEEK-BEEF BURGERS

Use only pasture-raised, 100 percent grass-fed beef, which has better essential fatty acid ratios and no added hormones or antibiotics. Leeks look like overgrown green onions and, like green onions, improve liver detoxification and add fiber, antioxidants, and chlorophyll.

1 large leek, chopped (about 2 cups)

1/3 cup olive oil

1 teaspoon dulse (seaweed)

1/2 teaspoon salt

1 pound ground beef (95 percent lean)

Lettuce leaves, sliced tomato, and sliced pickle (optional)

1. To clean the leek, trim any wilted ends and split the leek lengthwise. Submerge the leek pieces in a bowl of water and rub away any soil accumulated in the layers, especially where the green meets the white parts. Remove them from the water and drain.

2. In a food processor, blend the leek, olive oil, dulse, and salt into a thick paste. Add the ground beef and mix completely. If you don't have a food processor, finely mince the leek and mix it, the oil, dulse, salt, and ground beef with your hands.

3. Shape this mixture into 5 patties and cook in an oiled iron skillet on medium heat until browned on both sides (about 15 minutes total).

4. Garnish with lettuce, sliced tomato, and pickle if desired. Serve with steamed vegetables and a green salad.

Makes 5 servings, each containing 271 calories, 20 grams of protein, 19 grams of fat, 5 grams of carbohydrate, and 1 gram of fiber

DESSERTS

Making our own desserts lets us not only control the quality of the ingredients, but also appreciate the care that goes into making them. We may be more satisfied eating fewer sweets when they are made from whole foods instead of nutrient-depleting chemicals and refined sugars. These desserts are free of refined sugar, but still contain fruit and their natural sugars. Enjoy them on special occasions if you aren't experiencing acute IBS symptoms.

These desserts are sweetened naturally with fruit, honey, stevia, or all of these, the most traditional sweetening ingredients.

FLAX ICING

This is a high-fiber way to moisten and decorate a healthy cake.

1/4 cup flaxseeds

1/4 teaspoon cardamom powder

1/4 teaspoon coriander powder

1/4 teaspoon cinnamon powder

1/4 teaspoon stevia green-leaf powder

1 cup winter squash, baked, peeled, and cubed

1 cup warm water (just enough to get a thick, but spreadable, consistency

1/2 cup blueberries, raspberries, or blackberries (optional)

1. In a dry blender, finely grind the flaxseeds. Add the spices, stevia, and squash, and blend with the water until smooth.

2. Spread on Banana-Almond Bread (or Muffins) (recipe follows), and allow it to thicken for 10 to 20 minutes. Garnish with fresh berries, if desired.

Makes enough to cover a 9 x 12-inch cake or 12 muffins, each serving containing 19 calories, 1 gram of protein, 1 gram of fat, 2 grams of carbohydrate, and 1 gram of fiber

BANANA-ALMOND BREAD (OR MUFFINS)

Your whole family will love this moist, rich bread, plus it travels well. You can make your own almond or pumpkin seed flour in a food processor or buy it at most health food stores. Bob's Red Mill is a good brand.

2 1/2 cups organic almonds or pumpkin seeds

1 teaspoon baking soda

3 large organic eggs

2 very ripe bananas

1/2 teaspoon stevia green-leaf powder

1 tablespoon apple cider vinegar or lemon juice

1/4 cup melted organic coconut oil or coconut milk

Water to adjust batter thickness, approximately 1/2 cup

1. Preheat oven to 350°F.

2. If creating a loaf bread, oil a 9 x 12-inch baking dish. For muffins, line a cupcake tin with cupcake liners.

3. In a food processor, grind the almonds or pumpkin seeds into a fine powder.

4. Leaving the almond or pumpkin seed flour in the processor, slowly blend in the other ingredients in the order listed. Add the water last, adding just enough to make the batter slightly thicker than pancake batter.

5. Pour into the baking dish or cupcake liners, leaving a 1/2-inch space at the top to allow for expansion. Bake at 350°F for 20 to 30 minutes, until the surface springs back when pressed or a toothpick comes out clean.

6. The bread may flatten a bit after it cools, but this won't affect the taste. Serve as is, or frost with Flax Icing (previous page).

Makes 12 servings, each containing 184 calories, 6 grams of protein, 15 grams of fat, 9 grams of carbohydrate, and 3 grams of fiber

COCONUT-CAROB CANDIES

This is a great chocolate substitute, because it contains only two ingredients and no added sugar or artificial sweeteners. If you're addicted to chocolate, I can't guarantee this will *completely* replace it, but it will help if sugar or chocolate is your nemesis. Carob (St. John's Bread) is the bean pod of a kind of locust tree. Naturally sweet and alkalinizing, roasted carob is also rich in tannins, calcium, and iron. It's astringent as well, and has been used to help control diarrhea. Unlike cocoa, it doesn't contain caffeine or oxalic acid. Carob's tannins can inhibit fungus and microbes but also protein absorption, so limit it in children's diets.

Coconut oil melts at or above 77°F and contains medium-chain triglycerides, which the body preferentially uses for energy instead of storage. Many people have found that a small serving of a fat-rich treat, such as this one, satisfies the appetite and signals the end of a meal. Consuming small amounts of coconut oil a half hour before a meal may reduce your appetite and prevent overeating (Enig and Fallon 2005).

These candies are simple to make.

1 cup organic coconut oil, melted

1/2 cup roasted carob powder

1. Pour the oil into a 1-quart glass measuring cup. Add the carob powder and mix them together, using a whisk to get rid of all lumps.

2. Pour the mixture into ice cube trays, filling each cube space 1/4 to 1/2 full.

3. Chill in the freezer to harden. When the candies have solidified, pop them out of the tray and store them in a jar in the refrigerator or freezer. Enjoy with caution: they can be habit forming, but are also very satisfying.

Variation 1: Add chopped nuts or dried fruit, and pour out onto a cookie tray lined with parchment paper. Chill in the freezer as mentioned. Once candies have hardened, break them into bite-sized pieces.

Variation 2: Place 1 teaspoon of coconut-carob liquid in each unit of the ice cube tray and chill. Place a small dab (1/2 teaspoon) of nut butter, nuts, or dried fruit in each unit and cover with more coconut-carob liquid. Chill again and enjoy.

Makes about 24 bite-sized pieces, each serving (3 teaspoon-sized pieces without nuts) containing 132 calories, 0.3 grams of protein, 14.2 grams of fat, 5.7 grams of carbohydrate, and 2.5 grams of fiber, plus a rich supply of antimicrobial medium-chain triglycerides

BANANA-CASHEW PUDDING

This pudding is so yummy, you'll want to eat a lot of it, and so rich, you can't. A little goes a long way. You can also freeze it as a wonderful dairy-free, sugar-free ice cream substitute.

1/4 cup raw organic cashews, soaked for 1 hour

1/4 cup water

1 teaspoon vanilla extract (optional)

1 to 2 very ripe bananas

4 raspberries

1. Soak cashews for 1 hour or more in enough water to cover them completely.

2. Drain the cashews, put them in a blender, and add the fresh water. Add the vanilla if desired. Blend the mixture until very smooth. If you need to add more water to get everything to blend, add it slowly by the tablespoon so there's just enough liquid to blend completely. *Variation*: Blend in 1 to 2 tablespoons of carob powder and add more water, if needed for blending.

3. Add the bananas and continue blending until everything is thoroughly mixed. The mixture should be very thick.

4. Scoop the pudding into serving bowls. Garnish with raspberries and serve, or freeze the pudding in a small container with a lid and serve as you would gelato or ice cream.

Makes about 4 (1/2-cup) servings, each containing 133 calories, 3 grams of protein, 6 grams of fat, 18 grams of carbohydrates, and 2.2 grams of fiber

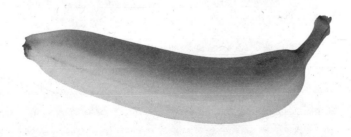

FRUIT COMPOTE

Apples inhibit the growth of disease-producing bacteria in the digestive tract (Wood 1999). Both apples and pears are moistening and help relieve constipation. The warming spices in this recipe make it a good choice on a cold winter night. Granny Smith and pippin apples are tart and complement the sweetness of the pears. Bartlett, Bosc, Anjou, and Asian pears have slightly different textures and tastes from one another. Try different varieties of apples, pears, and spices to see which you prefer. Top with flaxseeds or Cashew Cream (page 170).

1/2 tablespoon coconut oil

1 apple, sliced

1 pear, sliced

1/4 teaspoon cinnamon, ground

1/4 teaspoon cardamom, ground (optional)

1/4 teaspoon coriander, ground (optional)

1/8 teaspoon ginger, ground (optional)

1/8 teaspoon nutmeg, ground (optional)

1 to 2 tablespoons water (optional)

Flaxseeds or Cashew Cream (page 170) (optional)

1. In a small saucepan, melt the coconut oil. Add the sliced fruit and the cinnamon and other spices, as desired. Simmer on low heat, stirring occasionally. Add water, if needed, to prevent the fruit from sticking to the pan.

2. When the fruit is soft and the liquid is mostly gone, remove it from the heat and serve it hot, topped with flaxseeds or cashew cream.

Serves 2, each serving containing 104 calories, 1 gram of protein, 4 grams of fat, 19 grams of carbohydrate, and 5 grams of fiber

NUTTY CARROT CAKE

The carrots make this intensely rich cake a good source of beta-carotene. Use a Bundt pan and frost with Flax Icing (page 160) if desired.

3 cups brown rice flour

1 tablespoon baking soda

2 teaspoons baking powder

2 teaspoons cinnamon

1/2 teaspoon stevia green-leaf powder

1/2 teaspoon mineral salt or sea salt

4 large eggs

1 cup melted coconut oil

1/2 cup honey

3 cups organic carrots (approximately 1 pound), grated

1/4 cup lemon juice

1/2 cup walnuts, chopped

1/2 cup flaxseeds, whole

1. Preheat oven to 350° F. Lightly grease a Bundt pan or a 9 x 12-inch baking pan with coconut oil.

2. In a medium bowl, combine the flour, baking soda and powder, cinnamon, stevia, and salt.

3. In a separate, large mixing bowl, beat together the eggs, oil, and honey. Add the dry ingredients to the egg mixture and stir thoroughly.

4. Add the carrots, lemon juice, nuts, and flaxseeds. Mix and immediately pour into the pan.

5. Bake at 350°F for 45 to 60 minutes, until a toothpick comes out clean.

Makes 16 servings, each containing 336 calories, 5 grams of protein, 20 grams of fat, 36 grams of carbohydrate, 4 grams of fiber, plus 70 percent of your daily beta-carotene needs

SWEET POTATO PIE

A crowd pleaser, this simple pie is great for any holiday. Also called yams in America, sweet potatoes are in season in fall and winter. Choose yams with a firm, orange flesh, often called garnet yams or Japanese yams. If you use a hand mixer to blend the filling, remove the peels and use them in the Vegetable Stock recipe (page 142). I use a food processor and prefer to leave the peels on, because the peel contains most of the vitamins, minerals, and fiber. This crust is a grain-free version of a crumb crust, but much tastier. The secret is soaking the nuts ahead of time to eliminate any bitterness, and re-drying them.

Nutty Crust:

1 1/2 cups pecans or walnuts, soaked and re-dried (see recipe for Soaked, Dried Nuts or Seeds, page 110)

2 tablespoons melted coconut oil

1/2 teaspoon cinnamon

1/4 teaspoon stevia green-leaf powder

Sweet Potato Filling:

2 pounds garnet sweet potatoes

3/4 cup melted coconut oil

1/4 cup melted coconut cream concentrate or coconut milk

1 to 1 1/2 tablespoons pumpkin pie spice

1. Preheat the oven to 350°F. To make the filling, bake the sweet potatoes for 1 hour at 350°F, until soft. Let them cool so you can handle them and cut them into chunks.

2. To make the crust, coarsely grind the nuts in a food processor.

3. Melt the oil, and add the cinnamon and stevia.

4. In a small bowl, thoroughly mix the nuts with the melted oil–spice mixture, then split the crumbly mixture evenly into two 9-inch pie pans. With a spoon, press and flatten the crust against the sides of the pans until even and about 1/4-inch thick. Don't worry if the top edge of the crust is uneven.

5. If using a hand beater, peel the yams to blend the chunks smoothly. If using a blender or food processor, leave the peels on. Put the chunks into the food processor along with the coconut oil, coconut cream, and spices, and blend thoroughly until smooth. Stop the processor and push the mixture down around the edges to make sure it's completely blended.

6. Pour the filling gently into the crusts. Serve warm or at room temperature for optimal flavor. Garnish with Cashew Cream (page 170) or shavings of cold coconut cream concentrate for added decadence.

Makes two 9-inch pies, 8 pieces each, each piece containing 251 calories, 2 grams of protein, 20 grams of fat, 17 grams of carbohydrate, and 3 grams of fiber

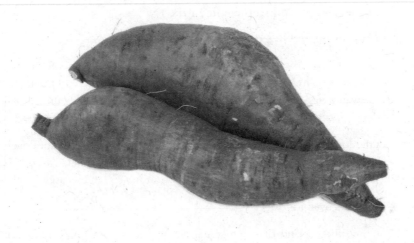

PUMPKIN PIE

What's Thanksgiving without pumpkin pie? This gluten-, dairy-, and sugar-free version allows nearly everyone to enjoy this seasonal treat. For a simpler crust, try using the nutty crust in the Sweet Potato Pie recipe (page 166).

Pie Crust:

2 cups organic buckwheat flour

1/2 cup cold coconut oil

1/2 cup cold water

Pumpkin Filling:

4 large eggs, beaten

12 ounces coconut milk, or 1/4 cup coconut cream concentrate (www.tropicaltraditions.com) blended with 1 cup warm water

3 3/4 cups organic pumpkin, baked, peeled, and puréed (about 1 1/2 pounds) or 2 (15-ounce) cans organic pumpkin purée

1 tablespoon pumpkin pie spice mix

1/2 teaspoon stevia green-leaf powder

1. To make the pie crust, in a medium bowl, cut the cold coconut oil into the flour with two knives or a pastry cutter until the oil is the size of peas. Mix in the water with a fork until just moistened, and knead briefly until a ball of dough forms.

2. Cut the dough in half and place each half in a 9-inch pie pan. Flatten the dough evenly in the pan with the back of a spoon or your fingers, about 1/8- to 1/4-inch thick. Flute the edges of the dough with your fingers, and set aside.

3. Preheat the oven to 350°F.

4. For the filling, blend or stir together the eggs, coconut milk, pumpkin, spice, and stevia in a large bowl or blender. Pour into pie shells.

5. Bake for 1 hour at 350°F or until firm in the center.

6. Serve plain or with Cashew Cream as topping (page 170).

Makes two 9-inch pies, 8 pieces each, each piece containing 237 calories, 5 grams of protein, 13 grams of fat, 29 grams of carbohydrate, and 7 grams of fiber

BLUEBERRY PIE

Excellent for summer parties, this no-bake pie is cool, light, refreshing, and loaded with fiber and antioxidants. The filling can also be served without the crust as a fruit gelatin, if desired. Try it using blackberries, raspberries, strawberries, or a mixture of these fruits.

You can use either gelatin powder or Pomona's Universal Pectin, a type of pectin that doesn't require added sugar and is activated by the calcium phosphate that comes with it. You mix the calcium phosphate with water to make calcium water. You can find it at health food stores or food co-ops (see pectin in Resources).

Make the nutty crust in the Sweet Potato Pie recipe (page 166). Reserve half of the crust recipe to use as a topping. Put the formed crust in the refrigerator to chill.

Berry Filling:

3/4 cup water

3 1/2 tablespoons unflavored gelatin (2 packets), or 1 tablespoon pectin powder and 4 teaspoons calcium water

1/4 cup lemon juice (juice of 3 lemons)

1 cup unsweetened applesauce or 1 large apple, chopped, cooked, and mashed

1/2 teaspoon cinnamon

4 cups organic fresh blueberries or berry mix (2 pints), or 16 ounces frozen organic blueberries

1. To make the filling, put the water, gelatin or pectin, lemon juice, applesauce or mashed apple, and cinnamon in a medium saucepan and heat to dissolve, stirring constantly.

2. Add the berries and mix together thoroughly. Remove the pan from the heat.

3. Pour the thickened fruit mixture into the crust. Garnish with the remaining crumb crust. Serve immediately or after chilling.

Makes one 9-inch pie or about 8 servings, each containing 238 calories, 3 grams of protein, 18 grams of fat, 21 grams of carbohydrate, and 5 grams of fiber

CASHEW CREAM

This dairy-free cream is sweet on its own, without any added sugar. Use it instead of commercial chemical concoctions. It's simple to make if you have a blender and plan ahead. (For more information on cashews, see the "Nut Milks" section of recipes, pages 94 and 95.)

1 cup organic raw cashews

1 cup water

1. In a blender, soak cashews for about 1 hour in enough water to cover them.

2. Drain the soaking water and replace it with 1 cup of fresh water. Blend until totally smooth.

Serve as a topping for any dessert or as you would whipped cream.

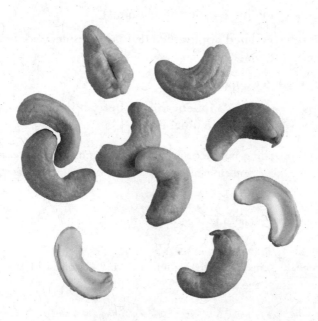

Resources

IBS INFORMATION

American College of Gastroenterology Functional Gastrointestinal Disorders Task Force. 2002. Evidence-based position statement on the management of irritable bowel syndrome in North America. *American Journal of Gastroenterology* 97 (Suppl. 11):S1–5.

National Digestive Diseases Information Clearinghouse, 2 Information Way, Bethesda, MD 20892-3570, 800-891-5389, http://digestive.niddk.nih.gov /ddiseases/pubs/ibs/ibs.pdf.

LABORATORIES FOR ALTERNATIVE TESTS

Diagnos-Techs, Inc., 6620 S. 192nd Place, Bldg. J, Kent, WA 98032, 800-878-3787, diagnostechs.com

Genova Diagnostics, 63 Zillicoa Street, Asheville, NC 28801, 800-522-4762, www.genovadiagnostics.com

The Great Plains Laboratory, Inc., 11813 W. 77th Street, Lenexa, KS 66214, 913-341-8949, www.greatplainslaboratory.com

Metametrix Clinical Laboratory, 3425 Corporate Way, Duluth, GA 30096, 800-221-4640, www.metametrix.com

Immuno Laboratories, Inc., 6801 Powerline Road, Fort Lauderdale, FL 33309, 800-231-9197, immunolabs.com

EnteroLab, 10875 Plano Road, Ste. 123, Dallas, TX 75238, 972-686-6869, www .enterolab.com

FOOD ALLERGY INFORMATION

Taylor, F., J. Krohn, and E. M. Larson. 2000. *Allergy Relief and Prevention: A Doctor's Complete Guide to Treatment and Self-Care*. 3rd ed. Point Roberts, WA: Hartley and Marks Publishers

TESTS TO RULE OUT CELIAC DISEASE

Obtain such tests through your licensed practitioner.

- Antibody blood tests: anti-tissue transglutaminase (tTG-IgA), anti-endomysial antibodies (EMA), and total serum IgA to test for IgA deficiency

- HLA-DQ2 and HLA-DQ8 gene tests—blood tests

- Low calcium, vitamin B12, vitamin D—blood tests

- High stool fat and protein—stool test

- Biopsy of small intestine (probably unnecessary if all the above tests are positive or all are negative)

FOOD ADDITIVE INFORMATION

Center for Science in the Public Interest, cspinet.org/reports/chemcuisine.htm

Farlow, C. H. 2005. *Dying to Look Good: The Disturbing Truth About What's Really in Your Cosmetics, Toiletries, and Personal Care Products*. Escondido, CA: Kiss for Health Publishing: dyingtolookgood.com

PHYSICIAN REFERRALS

International Health Foundation, PO Box 3494, Jackson, TN 38303, 901-423-5400

International College of Applied Kinesiology (ICAK) USA, referrals: 913-384-5336

Joan Margaret, DC, Chiropractor and Applied Kinesiologist, 6536 Telegraph Ave., Suite A102, Oakland CA 94609, 510-658-9066

Len Saputo, MD, 3799 Mt. Diablo Boulevard, Lafayette, CA 94549, 925-937-9550

The American Association of Naturopathic Physicians, naturopathic.org

American Holistic Medical Association, holisticmedicine.org

Candida research e-mail list, e-mail: listproc@stonebow.otago.ac.nz

Richard Cannon, Ph.D. (Candida research e-mail list administrator), Department of Oral Biology and Oral Pathology, University of Otago, PO Box 647, Dunedin, New Zealand

SEAWEEDS

Gualala Seaweed Products, PO Box 314, Gualala, CA 95445, 707-884-3726, e-mail: gualalaseaweedproducts.com

Mendocino Sea Vegetable Company, PO Box 455, Philo, CA 95466, 707-895-2996, seaweed.net

Ocean Harvest Sea Vegetable Company, PO Box 1719, Mendocino, CA 95460, 707-937-0637, ohsv.net

Rising Tide Sea Vegetables, PO Box 1914, Mendocino, CA, wholesale orders: 707-964-5663, loveseaweed.com

FERMENTED FOODS

Cultured (organic raw sauerkrauts and other fermented vegetables), 800 Bancroft Way, Berkeley, CA 94702, 510-540-5185

G.E.M. Cultures (starters for yogurt, kefir, and other ferments), 30301 Sherwood Rd., Ft. Bragg, CA 95437, 707-964-2922

South River Miso Company, 888 Shelburne Falls Rd., Conway, MA 01341, 413-369-4057, www.southrivermiso.com

PECTIN

Workstead Industries (Pomona's Universal Pectin), PO Box 1083, Greenfield, MA 01302, 413-772-6816, e-mail: info@pomonapectin.com, pomonapectin.com

PREFERRED SUPPLEMENT SOURCES

Metagenics, 100 Avenida La Pata, San Clemente, CA 92673, 800-692-9400, www.metagenics.com

Thorne Research, Inc., PO Box 25, Dover, ID 83825, 208-263-1337, e-mail: info@thorne.com, thorne.com

Standard Process, 1200 W. Royal Lee Drive, Palmyra, WI 53156, 800-558-8740, www.standardprocess.com

RELAXATION AIDS AND INFORMATION
Relaxation Products

Biodot of Indiana, Inc., PO Box 1207, Bedford, IN 47421, 800-272-2340, e-mail: biodot@hpcisp.com, www.biodots.net

The Journey to Wild Divine, Wild Divine, 2495 Truxtun Road, Bldg. 28, Ste. 208, San Diego, CA 92106, 866-594-9453, www.wilddivine.com/meditation -products.html

Relaxation Books

Benson, H., and M. Z. Klipper. 1975. *The Relaxation Response.* New York: HarperTorch

Davis, M., E. R. Eshelman, and M. McKay. 1995. *The Relaxation and Stress Reduction Workbook,* 4th ed. Oakland, CA: New Harbinger Publications

Stoll, W. 1996. *Saving Yourself from the Disease-Care Crisis.* Panama City, FL: Sunrise Health Coach Publications

TRADITIONAL FOOD INFORMATION

Price-Pottenger Nutrition Foundation, 7890 Broadway, Lemon Grove, CA 91945, 800-366-3748, info@ppnf.org

The Weston A. Price Foundation, 4200 Wisconsin Ave. NW, Washington, DC 20016, 202-363-4394, www.westonaprice.org

Three Stone Hearth (community supported kitchen, worker owned cooperative), 1581 University Ave., Berkeley, CA 94703, 510-981-1334, www .threestonehearth.com

SQUATTING PLATFORMS

Welles Step, www.juicing.com/wellesstep.htm

Lillipad Squat Toilet platform, lillipad.co.nz

RECOMMENDED READING

Adams, P. F., G. E. Hendershot, and M. A. Marano. 1999. Current estimates from the National Health Interview Survey, 1996. *National Center for Health Statistics: Vital and Health Statistics* 10 (200):1–203

Aihara, H. 1986. *Acid and Alkaline*. Oroville, CA: George Ohsawa Macrobiotic Foundation

Appleton, N. 1996. *Lick the Sugar Habit*. New York: Avery Publishing Group

Blanchard, K., and M. A. Brill. 2004. *What Your Doctor May Not Tell You About Hypothyroidism: A Simple Plan for Extraordinary Results*. New York: Warner Books

Bland, J. S., and S. H. Benum. 1999. *Genetic Nutritioneering: How You Can Modify Inherited Traits and Live a Longer, Healthier Life*. Lincolnwood, IL: Keats

Centers for Disease Control and Prevention (CDC). 2009. *Fourth national report on human exposure to environmental chemicals*. Atlanta, GA: CDC. www.cdc.gov /exposurereport

Dufty, W. 1975. *Sugar Blues*. New York: Warner Books

Erasmus, U. 1993. *Fats That Heal, Fats That Kill: The Complete Guide to Fats, Oils, Cholesterol, and Human Health*. 2nd ed. Burnaby, BC, Canada: Alive Books

Gottschall, E. G. 1994. *Breaking the Vicious Cycle: Intestinal Health Through Diet*. Baltimore, ON, Canada: Kirkton Press

Houghton, L. A., D. J. Heyman, and P. J. Whorwell. 1996. Symptomatology, quality of life, and economic features of irritable bowel syndrome: The effect of hypnotherapy. *Alimentary Pharmacology and Therapeutics* 10 (1):91–95

Katz, S. E. 2003. *Wild Fermentation: The Flavor, Nutrition and Craft of Life-Culture Foods*. White River Junction, VT: Chelsea Green

Nichols, T. W., and N. Faas. 1999. *Optimal Digestion: New Strategies for Achieving Digestive Health*. New York, NY: HarperCollins

Potts, B. 1988. *Witches Heal: Lesbian Herbal Self-Sufficiency*. 2nd ed. Ann Arbor, MI: DuReve Publications

Schmid, R. F. 1997. *Traditional Foods Are Your Best Medicine: Improving Health and Longevity with Native Nutrition*. Rochester, VT: Healing Arts Press

References

Accum, F. 1820. *A Treatise on Adulterations of Food and Culinary Poisons*. Philadelphia: Abraham Small. In Project Gutenberg, 2006, e-book 19031, gutenberg.org /files/19031/19031-h/19031-h.htm. July 2009.

Affenito, S. G. 2007. Breakfast: A missed opportunity. *Journal of the American Dietetic Association* 107 (4):565–69.

American College of Gastroenterology Functional Gastrointestinal Disorders Task Force. 2002. Evidence-based position statement on the management of irritable bowel syndrome in North America. *American Journal of Gastroenterology* 97 (Suppl. 11):S1–5.

Amira, S., S. Soufane, and K. Gharzouli. 2005. Effect of sodium fluoride on gastric emptying and intestinal transit in mice. *Experimental and Toxicologic Pathology* 57 (1):59–64.

Antico, A., R. Soana, L. Clivio, and R. Baioni. 1989. Irritable colon syndrome in intolerance to food additives. [In Italian.] *Minerva dietologica e gastroenterologica* 35 (4):219–24.

Avena, N. M., P. Rada, and B. G. Hoebel. 2008. Evidence for sugar addiction: Behavioral and neurochemical effects of intermittent, excessive sugar intake. *Neuroscience and Biobehavioral Reviews* 32 (1):20–39.

Ball, G. F. M. 2006. *Vitamins in Foods: Analysis, Bioavailability, and Stability*. Boca Raton, FL: CRC Press.

Bauman, E. 2008. *Eating for Health: Your Guide to Optimal Health and Vitality*. Penngrove, CA: Bauman College Press

Benbrook, C., X. Zhao, J. Yáñez, N. Davies, and P. Andrews. 2008. New evidence confirms the nutritional superiority of plant-based organic foods. *State of Science Review: Critical Issue Report*, March, 1–50.

Blanchard, K., and M. Abrams Brill. 2004. *What Your Doctor May Not Tell You About Hypothyroidism: A Simple Plan for Extraordinary Results*. New York: Warner Books.

Bland, J. S., and S. H. Benum. 1997. *The 20-Day Rejuvenation Diet Program*. New Canaan, CT: Keats Publishing.

Block, G. 2004. Foods contributing to energy intake in the US: Data from NHANES III and NHANES 1999–2000. *Journal of Food Composition and Analysis* 17 (3–4):439–47.

Bolen, B. B. 2009. What Is IBS? About.com, http://ibs.about.com/od/whatisib1/a/IBS.htm, June 22 (accessed November 2, 2009).

Brostoff, J., and L. Gamlin. 2000. *Food Allergies and Food Intolerance: The Complete Guide to Their Identification and Treatment*. Rochester, VT: Healing Arts Press.

Brynie, F. H. 2002. *101 Questions About Food and Digestion That Have Been Eating at You—Until Now*. Brookfield, CT: Twenty-First Century Books.

Camilleri, M. 2008. Probiotics and irritable bowel syndrome: Rationale, mechanisms, and efficacy. *Journal of Clinical Gastroenterology* 42 (Suppl. 3, pt. 1):S123–25.

Cannon, W. B. 1915. *Bodily Changes in Pain, Hunger, Fear, and Rage: An Account of Recent Researches into the Function of Emotional Excitement*. New York: D. Appleton and Company.

Clarke, L., J. McQueen, A. Samid, and A. R. Swain. 1996. Dietitians Association of Australia review paper: The dietary management of food allergy and food intolerance in children and adults. (PDF). *Australian Journal of Nutrition and Dietetics* 53 (3):89–98.

Colantuoni, C., P. Rada, J. McCarthy, C. Patten, N. M. Avena, A. Chadeayne, and B. G. Hoebel. 2002. Evidence that intermittent, excessive sugar intake causes endogenous opioid dependence. *Obesity Research* 10 (6):478–88.

Collins, S. M. 1994. Irritable bowel syndrome could be an inflammatory disorder. *European Journal of Gastroenterology and Hepatology* 6 (6):478–82.

Cordain, L., S. B. Eaton, A. Sebastian, N. Mann, S. Lindeberg, B. A. Watkins, J. H. O'Keefe, and J. Brand-Miller. 2005. Origins and evolution of the Western diet: Health implications for the 21st century. *American Journal of Clinical Nutrition* 81 (2):341–54.

Crewe, J. E. 1929. Raw milk cures many diseases. *Certified Milk*, January, 3–6.

Crinnion, W. J. 2000. Environmental medicine, part 4: Pesticides—Biologically persistent and ubiquitous toxins. *Alternative Medicine Review* 5 (5):432–47.

D'Mello, J. P. F. 2003. *Food Contaminants and Human Health*. Oxfordshire, UK: CAB International.

Davis, A. 1970. *Let's Eat Right to Keep Fit.* New York: Signet.

Davis, M., E. R. Eshelman, and M. McKay. 1995. The Relaxation and Stress Reduction Workbook. 4th ed. Oakland, CA: New Harbinger Publications.

DeCava, J. A. 2006. *The Real Truth About Vitamins and Antioxidants.* Fort Collins, CO: Selene River Press.

de Pomerai, D. I., B. Smith, A. Dawe, K. North, T. Smith, D. B. Archer, I. R. Duce, D. Jones, and E. P. Candido. 2003. Microwave radiation can alter protein conformation without bulk heating. *FEBS Letters* 543 (1–3):93–97.

Drettner, B. 1964. Vascular reactions on the intake of food and drink of various temperatures. *Acta oto-laryngologica* 57 (Suppl. 188):249–57.

Enig, M.G. 2000. *Know Your Fats: The Complete Primer for Understanding the Nutrition of Fats, Oils, and Cholesterol.* Silver Spring, MD: Bethesda Press.

Enig, M. G., and S. Fallon. 2005. *Eat Fat, Lose Fat: Lose Weight and Feel Great with the Delicious, Science-Based Coconut Diet.* New York: Penguin.

Faber, S., S. Rigden, and D. Lukaczer. 2005. The use of probiotics in the treatment of irritable bowel syndrome: Two case reports. *Alternative Therapies in Health and Medicine* 11 (4):60–62.

Fairley, K. J., R. Purdy, S. Kearns, S. E. Anderson, and B. J. Meade. 2007. Exposure to the immunosuppresant, perfluorooctanoic acid, enhances the murine IgE and airway hyperreactivity response to ovalbumin. *Toxicological Sciences* 97 (2):375–83.

Fallon, S., and M. G. Enig. 1999. *Nourishing Traditions: The Cookbook That Challenges Politically Correct Nutrition and the Diet Dictocrats.* Washington, DC: New Trends Publishing.

Farrer, K. T. H. 1987. *A Guide to Food Additives and Contaminants.* Nashville, TN: Parthenon Publishing Group.

Frassetto, L., R. C. Morris Jr., D. E. Sellmeyer, K. Todd, and A. Sebastian. 2001. Diet, evolution, and aging: The pathophysiologic effects of the post-agricultural inversion of the potassium-to-sodium and base-to-chloride ratios in the human diet. *European Journal of Nutrition* 40 (5):200–13.

Friel, P. 2006. Recent peer-reviewed research on serum IgG-based food allergy tests. *Townsend Letter for Doctors and Patients,* January.

Fujita, T., J. Tokunaga, and H. Inoue. 1971. *Atlas of Scanning Electron Microscopy in Medicine.* New York: Elsevier Publishing.

Gaby, A. R. 1998. The role of hidden food allergy/intolerance in chronic disease. *Alternative Medicine Review* 3 (2):90–100.

Galland, L. 1995. Leaky gut syndromes: Breaking the vicious cycle. HealthWorld Online. www.healthy.net/library/articles/galland/Leakygut.html.

Gates, D. 2006. *The Body Ecology Diet: Recovering Your Health and Rebuilding Your Immunity.* 9th ed. Atlanta, GA: Body Ecology Diet Publications.

Gittleman, A. L. 2001. *Guess What Came to Dinner: Parasites and Your Health*. Rev. ed. New York: Avery.

Goldberg, B., L. Trivieri, and J. W. Anderson. 2002. *Alternative Medicine: The Definitive Guide*. 2nd ed. Berkeley, CA: Celestial Arts.

Gottschall, E. G. 1994. *Breaking the Vicious Cycle: Intestinal Health Through Diet*. Baltimore, ON, Canada: Kirkton Press.

Gupte, S. 1975. Use of berberine in treatment of giardiasis. *American Journal of Diseases of Children* 129 (7):866.

Gyorgy, P. 1954. Vitamin B6 in human nutrition. *Journal of Clinical Nutrition* 2 (1):44–46.

Haas, E. M. 1992. *Staying Healthy with Nutrition: The Complete Guide to Diet and Nutritional Medicine*. Berkeley, CA: Celestial Arts.

Hampton, T. 2008. Sugar substitutes linked to weight gain. *Journal of the American Medical Association* 299 (18):2137–38.

Harvey, R. F. 1989. Individual and group hypnotherapy in treatment of refractory irritable bowel syndrome. *Lancet* 1 (8635):424–25.

Hobbs, C. 1992. *Foundations of Health: Healing with Herbs and Foods*. Capitola, CA: Botanica Press.

Hogg, M. 2006. Popularity of probiotics growing, but viable bacteria are lacking in some supplements. *Candida and Gut Dysbiosis News*, December 18.

Hudson, D. E., A. A. Dalal, and P. A. LaChance. 1985. Retention of vitamins in fresh and frozen broccoli prepared by different cooking methods. *Journal of Food Quality* 8 (1):45–50.

International Labour Organization 2006. *Your Health and Safety at Work: Chemicals in the Workplace*. http://actrav.itcilo.org/actrav-english/telearn/osh/kemi/ciwmain.htm.

Ishikawa, Y., T. Tokura, N. Nakano, M. Hara, F. Niyonsaba, H. Ushio, Y. Yamamoto, T. Tadokoro, K. Okumura, and H. Ogawa. 2008. Inhibitory effect of honeybee-collected pollen on mast cell degranulation in vivo and in vitro. *Journal of Medicinal Food* 11 (1):14–20.

Johnson, F. M. 2002. How many food additives are rodent carcinogens? *Environmental and Molecular Mutagenesis* 39 (1):69–80.

Joneja, J. V. 2004. *Digestion, Diet, and Disease: Irritable Bowel Syndrome and Gastrointestinal Function*. Piscataway, NJ: Rutgers University Press.

Jones, S. S. 1995. *The Main Ingredients of Health and Happiness*. Nevada City, CA. Dawn Publications.

Juven, B., Y. Henis, and B. Jacoby. 1972. Studies on the mechanism of the antimicrobial action of oleuropein. *Journal of Applied Bacteriology* 35 (4):559–67.

Kaneda, Y., T. Tanaka, and T. Saw. 1990. Effects of berberine, a plant alkaloid, on the growth of anaerobic protozoa in axenic culture. *Tokai Journal of Experimental and Clinical Medicine* 15 (6):417–23.

Katz, S. E. 2003. *Wild Fermentation: The Flavor, Nutrition, and Craft of Live-Culture Foods*. White River Junction, VT: Chelsea Green Publishing Company.

Kilkens, T. O., A. Honig, M. Maes, R. Lousberg, and R. J. Brummer. 2004. Fatty acid profile and affective dysregulation in irritable bowel syndrome. *Lipids* 39 (5):425–31.

Lemann Jr., J., E. J. Lennon, W. R. Piering, E. L. Prien Jr., and E. S. Ricanati. 1970. Evidence that glucose ingestion inhibits net renal tubular reabsorption of calcium and magnesium in man. *Journal of Laboratory and Clinical Medicine* 75 (4):578–85.

Loiselle, B. 1993. *The Healing Power of Whole Foods*. Nicholasville, KY: HealthWays Nutrition.

Longstreth, G. F., W. G. Thompson, W. D. Chey, L. A. Houghton, F. Mearin, and R. C. Spiller. 2006. Functional bowel disorders. *Gastroenterology* 130 (5):1480–91.

Martin, A. 2007. Poison used in China is found in U.S.-made animal feed. *New York Times*, May 31, Business section.

Marx, A. 1996. Parasites. *Explore!* 7 (4):41–4.

May, B., H. D. Kuntz, M. Kieser, and S. Köhler. 1996. Efficacy of a fixed peppermint oil / caraway oil combination in non-ulcer dyspepsia. *Arzneimittel Forschung (Drug Research)* 46 (12):1149–53.

Mearin, F., A. Balboa, X. Badía, E. Baró, E. Caldwell, M. Cucala, M. Díaz-Rubio, A. Fueyo, J. Ponce, M. Roset, and N. J. Talley. 2003. Irritable bowel syndrome subtypes according to bowel habit: Revisiting the alternating subtype. *European Journal of Gastroenterology and Hepatology* 15 (2):165–72.

Mercola, J., and K. D. Pearsall. 2006. *Sweet Deception: Why Splenda, NutraSweet, and the FDA May Be Hazardous to Your Health*. Nashville, TN: Thomas Nelson.

Millán, N., O. Brito, and P. Hevia. 1984. Nutritional quality of soybean proteins and casein, thermally damaged, and determined in vivo by an enzymatic method. [In Spanish.] *Archivos Latinoamericanos de nutrición* 34 (4):708–23.

Miller, S. B. 2007. IgG food allergy testing by ELISA/EIA: What do they really tell us? *Townsend Letter for Doctors and Patients*, October.

Morris, R. D., A. M. Audet, I. F. Angelillo, T. C. Chalmers, and F. Mosteller. 1992. Chlorination, chlorination by-products, and cancer: A meta-analysis. *American Journal of Public Health* 82 (7):955–63.

Mozaffarian, D., and E. B. Rimm. 2006. Fish intake, contaminants, and human health. *Journal of the American Medical Association* 296 (15):1885–99.

Murray, M. T. 1996. Encyclopedia of Nutritional Supplements: The Essential Guide for Improving Your Health Naturally. Rocklin, CA: Prima Health.

Murray, M. T., and J. Pizzorno. 1998. *Encyclopedia of Natural Medicine*. Rev. 2nd ed. Rocklin, CA: Prima Health.

Nakamura, T., T. J. Klopfenstein, D. J. Gibb, and R. A. Britton. 1994. Growth efficiency and digestibility of heated protein fed to growing ruminants. *Journal of Animal Science* 72 (3):774–82.

Nichols, T. W., and N. Faass, eds. 1999. Optimal Digestion: New Strategies for Achieving Digestive Health. New York: HarperCollins.

O'Bryan, T. 2008. Unlocking the secrets of gluten sensitivity: Implications for neurological, musculoskeletal, and immune health. Lecture at Metagenics Educational Programs, April 20, in Millbrae, CA.

Olden, K. W., ed. 1996. *Handbook of Functional Gastrointestinal Disorders.* New York: Marcel Dekker.

Park, P. K., and D. O. Cliver. 1997. Cutting boards up close. *Food Quality* 3 (22): 57–59.

Penttinen-Damdimopoulou, P. E., K. A. Power, T. T. Hurmerinta, T. Nurmi, P. T. van der Saag, and S. I. Mäkelä. 2009. Dietary sources of lignans and isoflavones modulate responses to estradiol in estrogen reporter mice. *Molecular Nutrition and Food Research* 53 (8):996–1006.

Pinton, P., J. P. Nougayrède, J. C. del Rio, C. Moreno, D. E. Marin, L. Ferrier, A. P. Bracarense, M. Kolf-Clauw, and I. P. Oswald. 2009. The food contaminant deoxynivalenol decreases intestinal barrier permeability and reduces claudin expression. *Toxicology and Applied Pharmacology* 237 (1):41–48.

Pitchford, P. 2002. *Healing with Whole Foods: Asian Traditions and Modern Nutrition.* 3rd ed. Berkeley, CA: North Atlantic Books.

Pollan, M. 2008. *In Defense of Food: An Eater's Manifesto.* New York: Penguin Press.

Pottenger, F.M. 1938. Clinical evidences of the value of raw milk. *Certified Milk* 3 (7):17–22.

Price, W. A. 1945. *Nutrition and Physical Degeneration.* La Mesa, CA: Price-Pottenger Nutrition Foundation.

Quig, D. W. 1998. Cysteine metabolism and metal toxicity. *Alternative Medicine Review* 3 (4):262–70.

Rabbani, G. H., T. Butler, J. Knight, S. C. Sanyal, and K. Alam. 1987. Randomized controlled trial of berberine sulfate therapy for diarrhea due to enterotoxigenic *Escherichia coli* and *Vibrio cholerae. Journal of Infectious Diseases* 155 (5):979–84.

Rabovsky, J., D. J. Judy, and W. H. Pailes. 1986. In vitro effects of straight-chain alkanes (n-hexane through n-dodecane) on rat liver and lung cytochrome P-450. *Journal of Toxicology and Environmental Health* 18 (3):409–21.

Rani, B., and N. Khetarpaul. 1998. Probiotic fermented food mixtures: Possible applications in clinical anti-diarrhoea usage. *Nutrition and Health* 12 (2):97–105.

Ravnskov, U. 2000. *The Cholesterol Myths: Exposing the Fallacy That Saturated Fat and Cholesterol Cause Heart Disease.* Washington, DC: New Trends Publishing.

Reuter, G. 2001. The *Lactobacillus* and *Bifidobacterium* microflora of the human intestine: Composition and succession. *Current Issues in Intestinal Microbiology* 2 (2):43–53.

Rudin, D., and C. Felix. 1996. *Omega-3 Oils: A Practical Guide*. Garden City Park, NY: Avery.

Saito, Y. A., P. Schoenfeld, and G. R. Locke III. 2002. The epidemiology of irritable bowel syndrome in North America: A systematic review. *American Journal of Gastroenterology* 97 (8):1910–15.

Sanders, D. S., M. J. Carter, D. P. Hurlstone, A. Pearce, A. M. Ward, M. E. McAlindon, and A. J. Lobo. 2001. Association of adult coeliac disease with irritable bowel syndrome: A case-control study in patients fulfilling ROME II criteria referred to secondary care. *Lancet* 358 (9292):1504–08.

Schmid, R. F. 1997. *Traditional Foods Are Your Best Medicine: Improving Health and Longevity with Native Nutrition*. Rochester, VT: Healing Arts Press.

———. 2009. *The Untold Story of Milk, Revised and Updated: The History, Politics, and Science of Nature's Perfect Food: Raw Milk from Pasture-Fed Cows*. Washington, DC: NewTrends Publishing.

Schreder, E. 2006. *Pollution in People: A Study of Toxic Chemicals in Washingtonians*. Toxic-Free Legacy Coalition Report. pollutioninpeople.org/results/download.

Schroeder, H. A. 1971. Losses of vitamins and trace minerals resulting from processing and preservation of foods. *American Journal of Clinical Nutrition* 24 (5):562–73.

Selye, H. 1956. *The Stress of Life*. New York: McGraw-Hill.

Senior, K. 1998. Chinese herbs calm irritable bowels. *Lancet* 352 (9140):1605.

Shahbazkhani, B., M. Forootan, S. Merat, M. R. Akbari, S. Nasserimoghadam, H. Vahedi, and R. Malekzadeh. 2003. Coeliac disease presenting with symptoms of irritable bowel syndrome. *Alimentary Pharmacology and Therapeutics* 18 (2):231–35.

Siebecker, A. 2005. Traditional bone broth in modern health and disease. Townsend Letter for Doctors and Patients 259–60 (2–3):74–81.

Simopoulos, A. P. 2002. The importance of the ratio of omega-6/omega-3 essential fatty acids. *Biomedicine and Pharmacotherapy* 56 (8):365–79.

Spiller, R. C., D. Jenkins, J. P. Thornley, J. Hebden, T. Wright, M. Skinner, and K. Neal. 2000. Increased rectal mucosal enteroendocrine cells, T lymphocytes, and increased gut permeability following acute *Campylobacter* enteritis and in post-dysenteric irritable bowel syndrome. *Gut* 47 (6):804.

Steinman, D., and R. M. Wisner. 1996. *Living Healthy in a Toxic World: Simple Steps to Protect You and Your Family from Everyday Chemicals, Poisons, and Pollution*. 1st ed. New York: Berkley Publishing Group.

Stoll, W. 1996. *Saving Yourself from the Disease-Care Crisis*. Panama City, FL: Sunrise Health Coach Publications.

Subbaiah, T. V., and A. H. Amin. 1967. Effect of berberine sulphate on *Entamoeba histolytica. Nature* 215 (5100):527–28.

Talley, N. J. 2006. Irritable bowel syndrome. *Internal Medicine Journal* 36 (11):724–28.

Trowbridge, J. P., and M. Walker. 1986. *The Yeast Syndrome: How to Help Your Doctor Identify and Treat the Real Cause of Your Yeast-Related Illness.* New York: Bantam Books.

USDA Sugar and Sweeteners Team, Market and Trade Economics Division, Economic Research Service. 2008. U.S. consumption of caloric sweeteners: Table 50—U.S. per capita caloric sweeteners estimated deliveries for domestic food and beverage use, by calendar year. Washington, DC: United States Department of Agriculture (USDA). ers.usda.gov/briefing/sugar /data.htm#other (accessed April 30, 2009).

Vanderhoof, J. A., D. B. Whitney, D. L. Antonson, T. L. Hanner, J. V. Lupo, and R. J. Young. 1999. *Lactobacillus GG* in the prevention of antibiotic-associated diarrhea in children. *Journal of Pediatrics* 135 (5):564–68. '

Waxman, D. 1988. The irritable bowel: A pathological or a psychological syndrome? *Journal of the Royal Society of Medicine* 81 (12):718–20.

Whitehead, W. E., O. Palsson, and K. R. Jones. 2002. Systematic review of the comorbidity of irritable bowel syndrome with other disorders: What are the causes and implications? *Gastroenterology* 122 (4):1140–56.

WHO Task Group on Environmental Health Criteria for Principles for Modelling Dose-Response for the Risk Assessment of Chemicals. 2009. *Principles for Modelling Dose-Response for the Risk Assessment of Chemicals.* Environmental Health Criteria series, no. 239. Geneva, Switzerland: World Health Organization International Programme on Chemical Safety.

Wood, R. 1999. *The New Whole Foods Encyclopedia: A Comprehensive Resource for Healthy Eating.* New York: Penguin Books.

Yudkin, J. 1972. *Sweet and Dangerous.* New York: Bantam Books.

Zhang, S. J., J. D. Bruton, A. Katz, and H. Westerblad. 2006. Limited oxygen diffusion accelerates fatigue development in mouse skeletal muscle. *Journal of Physiology* 572 (pt. 2):551–59.

Index

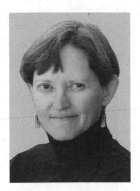**Laura J. Knoff, NC**, has been studying nutrition and biochemistry since 1975 and earned her nutrition consultant, nutrition educator, diet counselor, and nutrition instructor certificates from Bauman College in Penngrove, CA. She was a senior research associate at Lawrence Berkeley National Laboratory for eight years. She is now a registered professional member of the National Association of Nutritional Professionals and is board certified in holistic nutrition by that organization. She healed her own digestive disorders using whole foods, relaxation, and moderate exercise. Since 2000, she has taught prospective nutrition consultants at Bauman College in Berkeley, CA, and has a private practice at the Labrys Healthcare Circle in Oakland, CA.

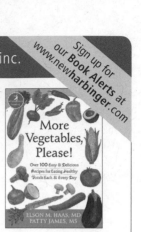
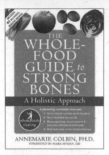
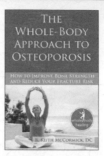
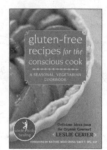
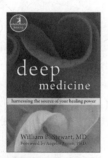
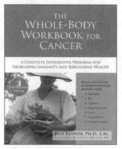